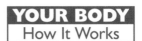

The Endocrine System

YOUR BODY How It Works

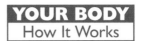

The Endocrine System

Lynette Rushton

Introduction by
Denton A. Cooley, M.D.
President and Surgeon-in-Chief
of the Texas Heart Institute
Clinical Professor of Surgery at the
University of Texas Medical School, Houston, Texas

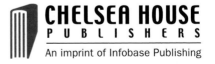

CHELSEA HOUSE
PUBLISHERS
An imprint of Infobase Publishing

The Endocrine System

Chelsea House
An imprint of Infobase Publishing
132 West 31st Street
New York NY 10001

Library of Congress Cataloging-in-Publication Data

Rushton, Lynette, 1954–
    The endocrine system / Lynette Rushton.
        p. cm. — (Your body, how it works)
Includes bibliographical references and index.
    ISBN 0-7910-7738-1
    1. Endocrine glands. 2. Hormones. I. Title. II. Series.
QP187.R938 2004
612.4—dc22   2004007198

Chelsea House books are available at special discounts when purchased in bulk quantities for businesses, associations, institutions, or sales promotions. Please call our Special Sales Department in New York at (212) 967-8800 or (800) 322-8755.

You can find Chelsea House on the World Wide Web at http://www.chelseahouse.com

Text and cover design by Terry Mallon

Printed in the United States of America

Bang 21C 10 9 8 7 6 5 4 3 2

This book is printed on acid-free paper.

All links and web addresses were checked and verified to be correct at the time of publication. Because of the dynamic nature of the web, some addresses and links may have changed since publication and may no longer be valid.

Table of Contents

Introduction

The human body is an incredibly complex and amazing structure. At best, it is a source of strength, beauty, and wonder. We can compare the healthy body to a well-designed machine whose parts work smoothly together. We can also compare it to a symphony orchestra in which each instrument has a different part to play. When all of the musicians play together, they produce beautiful music.

From a purely physical standpoint, our bodies are made mainly of water. We are also made of many minerals, including calcium, phosphorous, potassium, sulfur, sodium, chlorine, magnesium, and iron. In order of size, the elements of the body are organized into cells, tissues, and organs. Related organs are combined into systems, including the musculoskeletal, cardio-vascular, nervous, respiratory, gastrointestinal, endocrine, and reproductive systems.

Our cells and tissues are constantly wearing out and being replaced without our even knowing it. In fact, much of the time, we take the body for granted. When it is working properly, we tend to ignore it. Although the heart beats about 100,000 times per day and we breathe more than 10 million times per year, we do not normally think about these things. When something goes wrong, however, our bodies tell us through pain and other symptoms. In fact, pain is a very effective alarm system that lets us know the body needs attention. If the pain does not go away, we may need to see a doctor. Even without medical help, the body has an amazing ability to heal itself. If we cut ourselves, the blood clotting system works to seal the cut right away, and the immune defense system sends out special blood cells that are programmed to heal the area.

During the past 50 years, doctors have gained the ability to repair or replace almost every part of the body. In my own field of cardiovascular surgery, we are able to open the heart and repair its valves, arteries, chambers, and connections. In many cases, these repairs can be done through a tiny "keyhole" incision that speeds up patient recovery and leaves hardly any scar. If the entire heart is diseased, we can replace it altogether, either with a donor heart or with a mechanical device. In the future, the use of mechanical hearts will probably be common in patients who would otherwise die of heart disease.

Until the mid-twentieth century, infections and contagious diseases related to viruses and bacteria were the most common causes of death. Even a simple scratch could become infected and lead to death from "blood poisoning." After penicillin and other antibiotics became available in the 1930s and '40s, doctors were able to treat blood poisoning, tuberculosis, pneumonia, and many other bacterial diseases. Also, the introduction of modern vaccines allowed us to prevent childhood illnesses, smallpox, polio, flu, and other contagions that used to kill or cripple thousands.

Today, plagues such as the "Spanish flu" epidemic of 1918–19, which killed 20 to 40 million people worldwide, are unknown except in history books. Now that these diseases can be avoided, people are living long enough to have long-term (chronic) conditions such as cancer, heart failure, diabetes, and arthritis. Because chronic diseases tend to involve many organ systems or even the whole body, they cannot always be cured with surgery. These days, researchers are doing a lot of work at the cellular level, trying to find the underlying causes of chronic illnesses. Scientists recently finished mapping the human genome, which is a set of coded "instructions" programmed into our cells. Each cell contains 3 billion "letters" of this code. By showing how the body is made, the human genome will help researchers prevent and treat disease at its source, within the cells themselves.

The body's long-term health depends on many factors, called risk factors. Some risk factors, including our age, sex, and family history of certain diseases, are beyond our control. Other important risk factors include our lifestyle, behavior, and environment. Our modern lifestyle offers many advantages but is not always good for our bodies. In western Europe and the United States, we tend to be stressed, overweight, and out of shape. Many of us have unhealthy habits such as smoking cigarettes, abusing alcohol, or using drugs. Our air, water, and food often contain hazardous chemicals and industrial waste products. Fortunately, we can do something about most of these risk factors. At any age, the most important things we can do for our bodies are to eat right, exercise regularly, get enough sleep, and refuse to smoke, overuse alcohol, or use addictive drugs. We can also help clean up our environment. These simple steps will lower our chances of getting cancer, heart disease, or other serious disorders.

These days, thanks to the Internet and other forms of media coverage, people are more aware of health-related matters. The average person knows more about the human body than ever before. Patients want to understand their medical conditions and treatment options. They want to play a more active role, along with their doctors, in making medical decisions and in taking care of their own health.

I encourage you to learn as much as you can about your body and to treat your body well. These things may not seem too important to you now, while you are young, but the habits and behaviors that you practice today will affect your physical well-being for the rest of your life. The present book series, YOUR BODY: HOW IT WORKS, is an excellent introduction to human biology and anatomy. I hope that it will awaken within you a lifelong interest in these subjects.

Denton A. Cooley, M.D.
President and Surgeon-in-Chief
of the Texas Heart Institute
Clinical Professor of Surgery at the
University of Texas Medical School, Houston, Texas

1

Little Chemicals That Run the Body

The human body has an amazingly complex array of systems, such as the circulatory, digestive, and muscular systems, and each has important functions. In order to operate properly, all of the systems in the body must work together. This means that the body can regulate itself and that the various organs involved can communicate with each other.

The body has two systems for control and communication. One of these is the **nervous system**, which consists of the brain, spinal cord, and nerves. The nervous system receives and sends information through nerve cells (neurons) as electrical impulses. A nerve impulse can travel as fast as 100 meters/second (m/sec), and it targets a specific part of the body, such as a cell.

The other control system is the **endocrine system**. It consists of a group of organs called **endocrine glands**, which are located in various parts of the body. (These glands will be discussed individually in later chapters.) Endocrine glands release chemical messengers called **hormones** that travel through the blood. Because hormones take time to travel through the circulatory system, a response by the endocrine system will take much longer than one by the nervous system. However, hormones can travel everywhere in the body. For this reason, hormones control responses that do not need to be immediate, but have to be generalized and longer lasting. These responses include growth, reproduction, metabolic rate, blood glucose levels, and salt/water balance. Although the nervous and endocrine systems can be discussed separately, it is helpful to think of them as different aspects of a single control system. The nervous system is for immediate and specific responses, and the endocrine system is for slower, long-term, general types of responses.

Often, the two systems can produce the same response, and they may even utilize the same chemicals. The differences between the two systems involve how quickly the response occurs, and how long the response can be sustained. For example, both systems produce the chemical **epinephrine**, also called **adrenaline**. When a person is startled or frightened, the nervous system releases epinephrine from certain neurons that send information to internal organs. As a result, the person's heart rate increases, the brain becomes alert, blood flow to internal organs decreases, and more blood is sent to the muscles. This response, known as the **fight-or-flight response**, prepares the body for danger. The neurons have only a small amount of **neurotransmitter** (in this case, epinephrine) present at any given moment, and it is quickly depleted. This small amount is helpful for an instant response. The body, however, cannot maintain this aroused state for more than a few minutes on the neurons' supply of epinephrine alone. Each cell must produce more of the neurotransmitter before it can once again send a signal to the organ.

After a minute or two, the adrenal glands, the endocrine glands located near the kidneys, begin to release epinephrine. The response to this release of epinephrine will be the same as that produced by the nervous system. However, the adrenal glands can produce epinephrine continuously for days at a time. It is important to remember that the nervous system perceived the stress and sent the message to the adrenal glands in the first place. Neither system can function without the other. Table 1.1 details some of the differences between the two systems.

Table 1.1: Comparison of Nervous and Endocrine Systems

	Nervous System	Endocrine System
Mode of Information Transfer	Nerve impulse & neurotransmitter release at specific site	Hormone released into bloodstream
Receptor Location in Body	Internal & external	Internal
Effects:		
Location	Localized	Entire body
Targets	Nerve, gland, muscle cells	All tissues
Time for:		
Onset	Immediate (milliseconds)	Gradual (seconds to hours)
Duration	Short-term (milliseconds to minutes)	Long-term (minutes to days)
Recovery	Immediate (as soon as signal removed)	Slow (continues after signal removed)

Table 1.1 The endocrine and nervous systems cooperate to control the body. The nervous system is quick, short-term, and specific in its responses. The endocrine system works more slowly throughout the body and produces long-term effects.

SAVED FROM CERTAIN DEATH: LEONARD AND ELIZABETH

Insulin was the first hormone to be discovered and purified. It is produced by special cells in the pancreas and allows the cells of the body to absorb the sugar glucose (the cells' energy source) from the blood. Without enough insulin, the glucose remains in the blood and is excreted in the urine. When this occurs, the body's cells cannot import their food supply, and they starve.

Diabetes mellitus is the name given to the disorder caused by insufficient insulin in the body. It occurs when the body cannot make or process enough insulin to function properly. It has been known for thousands of years. Around 250 B.C., the Greeks used the word *diabetes* (meaning "to pass through"), because of the excessive thirst victims suffer and the large amount of urine they produce. The Latin *mellitus* ("honey") was added later, when it was discovered that the urine contained sugar. Weakness and weight loss ensue until the victim becomes emaciated. If left untreated, the victim eventually slips into a coma and dies, almost always within a year of diagnosis.

Even though the condition was known for centuries, an effective treatment was not discovered until much later. In 1921, two Canadian researchers, Frederick Banting and Charles Best (Figure 1.1), kept a severely diabetic dog alive by injecting it with extracts from the pancreas of other animals. They had discovered insulin. A biochemist named J. B. Collip began to work with them later to purify the insulin in their extracts and test it on humans. The first person to receive insulin was Leonard Thompson, a diabetic 14-year-old boy who weighed 64 pounds. Banting gave Leonard two injections of the insulin extract. Although Leonard's blood glucose levels dropped because the glucose was now entering his cells, he did not improve otherwise. In fact, he developed abscesses at the injection sites. Six weeks later, he was given a more purified injection. Within 24 hours, his blood glucose levels dropped from 520 mg/dL to 120 mg/dL, well within the range of normal. (The deciliter, dL, is one-tenth of a liter. It is the unit of volume typically used for blood concentrations.) Leonard quickly began to gain weight and strength as he continued to receive injections of the purified insulin prepared by Collip. The successful cure was reported in the *Toronto Daily Star* on

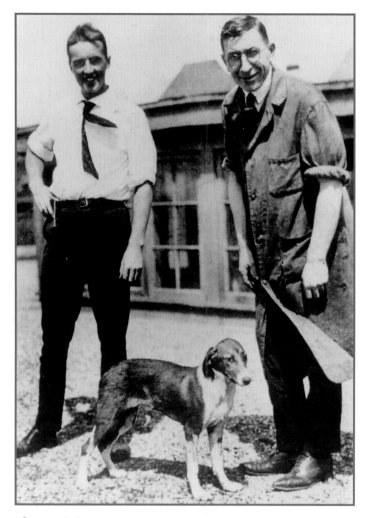

Figure 1.1 In 1921, Charles Best (left) and Frederick Banting (right) discovered insulin by working with diabetic dogs. Best and Banting are seen here with one of the dogs that received their insulin treatment.

March 22, 1922. The doctors were flooded with requests to treat dying children.

One of these children was Elizabeth Hughes, the daughter of New York Governor Charles Evans Hughes. Diagnosed with diabetes when she was 11, Elizabeth was being treated by her doctor through starvation, a treatment discovered in the late 19th century to keep diabetic patients alive.

Banting first saw Elizabeth just before her fifteenth birthday in 1922. She weighed 45 pounds, and she could barely walk. Her hair was thin and brittle. The insulin injections began to work immediately. Within one week, she was able to eat more than twice what she had been eating before without any glucose being excreted in her urine. After more than three months of treatment, Elizabeth weighed 105 pounds. Endocrinology, the study of hormones and their actions, had become a field of medicine, not just a research topic.

2

Hormones: What Are They and How Do They Work?

WHAT IS A HORMONE?

A hormone is a chemical that is carried by the blood to another part of the body, where it causes a particular response. Hormones, which are produced by endocrine glands, act on cells called "**target cells**." A target cell has protein molecules called receptors to which the hormone can attach. Each type of cell has a different set of proteins, so cells without the correct receptor molecules cannot respond to the hormone signal.

The term *hormone* was first used formally in 1905 by Ernest H. Starling. He used it to describe chemicals that were secreted inside the body by glands without ducts, as opposed to secretions that travel through tubes or ducts to reach their destination. The term *internal secretions* had been used until this time to refer to this phenomenon, but many researchers felt that the term was not precise enough to describe the growing number of chemical messengers that were being identified and isolated in the body. The word *hormone* was derived from the Greek verb *hormao*, which means "to excite" or "put into motion." Over the next 50 years, the definition of *hormone* developed into what it is currently: specific chemicals secreted from specific tissues into body fluid, usually blood. The hormones are then carried to another part of the body, where they have specific actions. Hormones are produced by cells and act on cells.

Currently, there are about 50 distinct chemicals in humans that have been identified as hormones. These messengers help the body carry out a number of vital functions. Some of these functions are long-term and ongoing, such as growth, development, and reproduction. Others are basic physiological operations, such as regulating blood glucose levels.

Hormones can be divided in two general chemical groups: steroids and nonsteroids. **Steroids**, which are **lipids**, include all of the **sex hormones** (testosterone, estrogens, and progesterone) and substances from the adrenal cortex, such as cortisone and 1,25-dihydroxycholecalciferol, a form of vitamin D. Because steroids are all derivatives of cholesterol, they are also called **sterols**. The differences between cholesterol and steroids lie in the side chains attached to the basic four-ring structure. If the structure of testosterone and 17-β-estradiol (an estrogen) are compared, the differences on the first ring (ring A) become apparent. Testosterone has a -CH_3, or methyl group, and a double-bonded oxygen, a carbonyl group, but estradiol has only a hydroxyl group (-OH). Figure 2.1 shows the structures of cholesterol, testosterone, and 17-β-estradiol.

Lipids are a large and diverse group of biological molecules. All lipids share one basic characteristic—they do not dissolve in water. Molecules that are not water-soluble are called **nonpolar**, or **hydrophobic** (water-hating). The structure of water molecules causes them to have one end slightly negatively charged and the other end slightly positively charged, similar to a battery, which has positive and negative ends. Substances that are **polar** will be attracted to water molecules, so they are called **hydrophilic** (water-loving). This chemical difference explains why some substances, such as salt and sugar, dissolve in water, but oil does not. Body fluids, including blood, are mostly water. A nonpolar molecule will not dissolve in water, so it will not readily enter or travel through body fluids. Lipids must use special

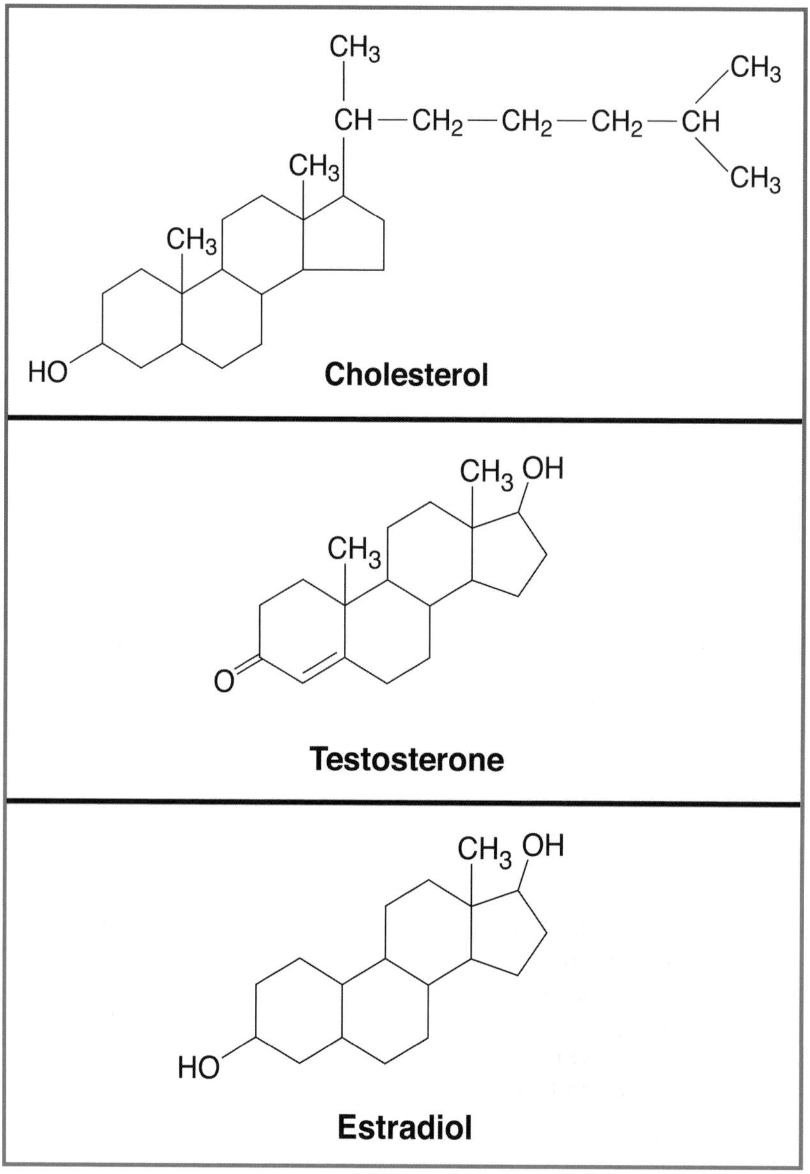

Figure 2.1 This diagram shows three common steroids. Cholesterol (top) is a component of cell membranes and is the basic molecule from which all other steroids are derived. Testosterone (center) is the male sex hormone. Estradiol (bottom) is one of the female sex hormones collectively called estrogens.

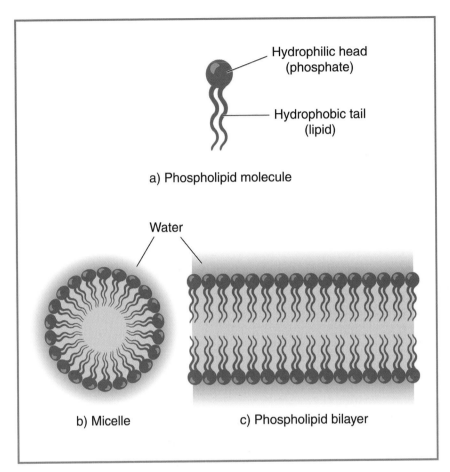

a) Phospholipid molecule

b) Micelle

c) Phospholipid bilayer

Figure 2.2 Phospholipids, illustrated here, consist of a phosphate ion and two long chains of hydrocarbons, called fatty acids, attached to a glycerol molecule. This gives them a hydrophobic (water-loving) head and hydrophobic (water-hating) tail. When placed in water, they form bubbles called micelles, or larger double layers that have their fatty acid tails tucked inside, away from the water.

transport systems to move through the blood. Because cell membranes are made primarily of lipids, all lipids can easily enter or leave cells.

Nonsteroid hormones include **proteins** (large molecules made up of chains of amino acids), such as insulin and growth hormone, and molecules called **amines**, such as thyroid hormone, which are modified amino acids. Proteins and amines are polar substances, meaning they are water-soluble (hydrophilic). They can easily enter and be carried by the blood plasma. Protein and amine molecules cannot cross the lipid cell membrane on their own to get into or out of cells.

As stated earlier, hormones travel through the blood and act on target cells. To understand how steroid and nonsteroid hormones travel through the body and act on these cells, it is necessary to learn some basic cell structure.

CELL STRUCTURE

All cells are surrounded by a membrane that is composed primarily of a double layer of lipid molecules called **phospholipids** (Figure 2.2). These are large, waterproof molecules that are similar to fat molecules. At one end of the molecule's structure, however, a polar phosphate group (PO_4^{-3}) has replaced one nonpolar group, making phospholipids both hydrophobic and hydrophilic. Phospholipids arrange themselves into two layers with the lipid tails in the middle and the phosphate heads on the surfaces in contact both with the watery external environment and the cytoplasm inside the cell that contains a great deal of water. Protein molecules are attached in, on, and through the bilayer. These proteins have many functions, including serving as receptors and channels for polar substances. Lipids, such as steroid molecules, can pass freely through the cell membrane (Figure 2.3).

SIGNAL TRANSDUCTION

Each target cell has a receptor protein for its specific hormone. The hormone molecule and its receptor attach to each other exclusively. Each molecule has a distinct three-dimensional shape. The receptor can be thought of as a lock and the

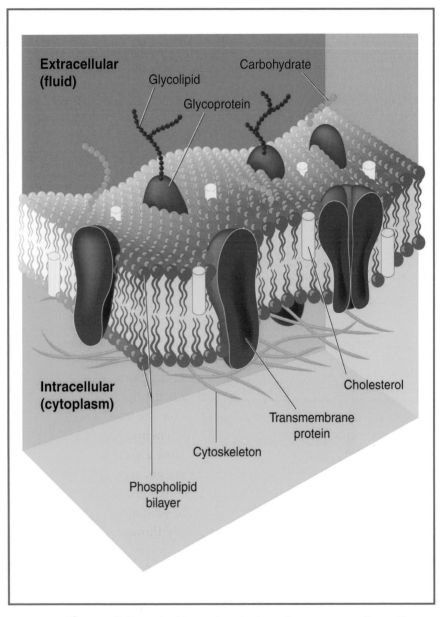

Figure 2.3 This illustration depicts the structure of a cell membrane. The phospholipids bilayer also contains cholesterol (yellow) and proteins (brown). The proteins serve as channels, receptors, and cell recognition sites.

hormone as the key that fits that lock. Once the hormone has attached to the receptor, the receptor changes, which in turn causes a change in the cell, a process called **signal transduction**. A chemical signal from outside the cell has brought about a response inside the cell.

Signal transduction occurs in three stages (Figure 2.4):

1. *Reception*: The hormone attaches to its receptor.

2. *Transduction*: The receptor protein alters and then produces a change or changes in the cell. If a sequence of changes occurs, the process is called a signal trans-duction pathway.

3. *Response*: Some behavior or property of the cell changes, such as a change in gene expression or activation of an enzyme.

Because protein hormones cannot enter a cell, their receptors must be located on the outside of the cell membrane. The receptor protein extends through the cell membrane and is attached to a signal protein on the inside of the cell. When a protein hormone molecule attaches to the receptor on the outside of the cell, it activates the signal inside the cell. Typically, the process will activate a series of molecules called a **cascade**.

The same hormone can produce different responses in different cells depending on the set of proteins the cell contains. The epinephrine of the fight-or-flight response causes heart muscle cells to contract more strongly, which increases the volume of blood pumped by the heart. When epinephrine attaches to a receptor on a liver cell, however, no contraction occurs because liver cells do not have contractile proteins. Liver cells, though, do have all the enzymes needed to store glucose in the form of a large branched polymer called **glycogen** and to split the glycogen back into glucose molecules. When epinephrine attaches to a receptor on a liver cell, it activates an enzyme that eventually results in the release of glucose into the bloodstream. Both the stronger heart contractions and increased blood glucose level help the person run away from danger.

When epinephrine attaches to the receptor on a liver cell membrane, 100 signal proteins (called **G proteins**) inside the cell are activated and, in turn, activate 100 enzyme molecules called **adenylate cyclase**. The adenylate cyclase catalyzes the conversion of ATP (adenosine triphosphate) to **cAMP** (cyclic adenosine monophosphate) many times. Each cAMP activates another enzyme called protein kinase A, and each molecule of protein kinase A activates several molecules of the next enzyme, phosphorylase kinase. This enzyme can activate up to 10 glycogen phosphorylase molecules, which then catalyze the breakdown of glycogen into glucose molecules.

A single hormone molecule can produce a large effect inside the cell by having multiple steps. For example, one molecule of epinephrine can cause a liver cell to release more than 100 million glucose molecules. Figure 2.4 shows the steps in the signal transduction process in a liver cell. The numbers are the approximate numbers of molecules activated or released at each step.

Because steroids and the tiny thyroid hormone can cross the cell membrane, the target cells for these hormones have the receptor proteins on the inside of the cell. When the hormone attaches to the receptor, the hormone-receptor complex becomes a transcription factor—a substance that enters the nucleus, attaches to the DNA, and controls the expression of a particular gene or genes. The gene may be turned on, causing a protein (an enzyme, for example) to be produced. Or the gene may be turned off, stopping the production of a protein. A transcription factor may regulate one or several genes. Steroid hormones will typically take longer to elicit a cell response than protein hormones do because they control protein synthesis. Protein hormones, in contrast, simply activate

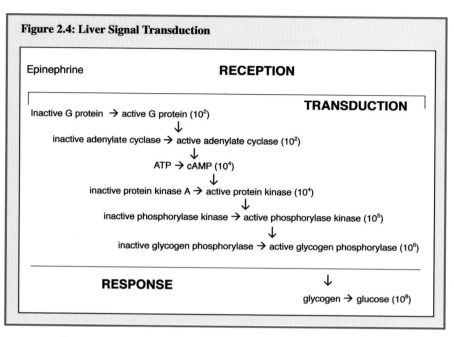

Figure 2.4 This figure shows the pathway by which epinephrine (adrenaline) increases blood glucose levels. At each step, a molecule is activated, which, in turn, starts the next step. The numbers refer to the number of molecules activated at each step. At the last step, glycogen—a storage form of glucose—splits to release glucose into the bloodstream. This process is called a cascade, in which a small signal (fewer than 100 epinephrine molecules) can cause a large response (10^8 glucose molecules).

molecules that are already present in the cell. Table 2.1 is a summary of the modes of hormone action.

CONTROL OF HORMONE RELEASE

To understand how the body controls the amount of hormones released, it is important first to understand some basic cell biology.

Homeostasis

For a cell to survive and function properly, it needs a certain environment. This environment can be thought of as the

Table 2.1: Summary of Hormone Actions

	Steroid & thyroid hormones	Protein hormones
Location of receptor	Cell cytoplasm or nucleus	Outer surface of cell membrane
Action pathway	Signal + hormone ↓ transcription factor ↓ DNA ↓ protein ↓ cell response	Signal + hormone ↓ active enzyme ↓ cell response

Table 2.1 Steroid and thyroid hormones enter cells and act by either stimulating or inhibiting gene expression. Protein hormones cannot enter cells, so they must act on cell membrane receptors. For this reason, protein hormones produce a response more quickly than steroids do.

fluid that surrounds every cell in the body. This fluid is called *interstitial* ("in the spaces") or *extracellular* fluid because it is outside of the cells (*exter* is Latin for "on the outside"). It consists mostly of water and contains dissolved substances, such as sodium, glucose, calcium, and proteins. The interstitial fluid comes from, and returns to, the blood plasma as the blood circulates through the body. The body must maintain nearly constant conditions of temperature, pH, and concentrations of glucose, sodium, and calcium in this fluid, or the cells will be adversely affected. This dynamic process of maintaining a constant internal environment is called **homeostasis**.

Homeostasis is typically achieved by a process called negative feedback. This process has three primary components: an error detector, a control or communication system, and a correcting mechanism. Controlling the temperature of a room using a thermostat is an example of negative feedback. The thermostat is set at the desired temperature (the set point). In the case of heating a room, if the temperature falls below the set point, a detector in the thermostat senses the drop and sends a message to the heat source. The furnace turns on, raising the temperature in the room. Once the temperature has reached the set point, the sensor in the thermostat responds and the furnace turns off. The body maintains homeostasis in a similar way. However, just as there are many ways to heat a house (a simple fire pit versus a computer-operated climate control system, for example), homeostatic mechanisms work in various ways.

The nervous and/or endocrine systems are typically the controlling aspects of negative feedback systems. The example of insulin and blood glucose described in Chapter 1 is a good example. When blood glucose levels rise, insulin is released. The insulin allows the cells to transport the glucose out of the blood, so the blood glucose levels drop. As blood glucose levels decrease, the amount of insulin being secreted also decreases. In this case, the internal environment directly controls hormone release. Some hormones are controlled by more complex pathways with many more steps in them, but the general mechanism is the same.

CONNECTIONS

Hormones are essential to the proper functioning of the human body. They control many functions, such as an individual's height, metabolic rate, and gender. Some hormones are released in response to the minute-by-minute changes in the body's interior, like blood glucose concentrations and insulin. Others are regulated over longer time periods—hours or even days or weeks. Some hormones allow our bodies to respond to the external environment (like the amount of daylight present). In that case, the information enters through the nervous system and is relayed to the endocrine system.

In the following chapters, you will learn about particular hormones and how they help individuals survive, reproduce, and maintain homeostasis. You will also learn about some of the most common endocrine disorders.

3

The Endocrine Organs

Hormones are secreted from organs called endocrine glands. These glands are called ductless glands because they do not connect to their target cells by tubes or ducts, but instead secrete their hormones directly into the bloodstream, which then carries the hormones throughout the body. The endocrine glands include organs, such as the thyroid and adrenal glands, whose only function is to secrete hormones. Other organs secrete hormones in addition to their other functions. For example, the pancreas produces many substances necessary for digestion as well as hormones that regulate blood glucose levels. Other organs, such as the kidneys and heart, have major functions that have nothing to do with hormones, but they secrete hormones as well. Figure 3.1 shows the location of the endocrine glands in the human body. This chapter will briefly examine each organ that produces hormones. Later chapters will look at certain processes controlled by hormones in more detail.

THE HYPOTHALAMUS AND PITUITARY GLAND

The **hypothalamus** is located near the center of the brain, above the brainstem and below the cerebrum (Figure 3.2). Its primary function is to maintain homeostasis, acting as the body's thermostat. The nervous system and endocrine system are truly integrated structurally and functionally in the hypothalamus. The hypothalamus receives chemical and nervous input about sight, sound, taste, smell, temperature, blood glucose concentrations, and salt/water balance. It also

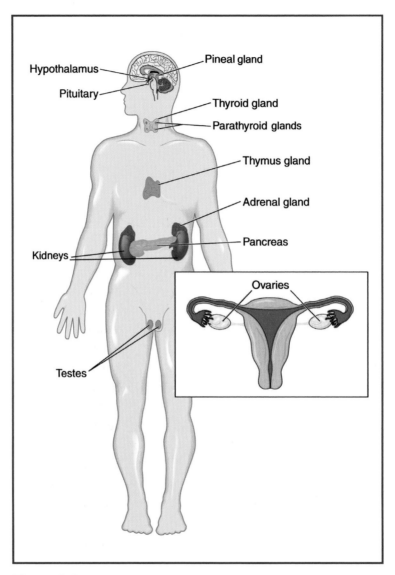

Figure 3.1 Each of the endocrine organs, illustrated here, produces one or more hormones. Some organs, like the pancreas and kidneys, also have other functions that are not related to hormones.

helps control hunger and thirst as well as mating and sexual behavior. The hypothalamus also has nervous input to functions such as the regulation of heart rate, blood pressure, and contractions of the urinary bladder.

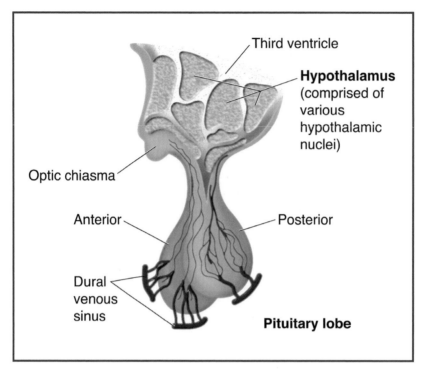

Third ventricle

Hypothalamus
(comprised of
various
hypothalamic
nuclei)

Optic chiasma

Anterior

Posterior

Dural
venous
sinus

Pituitary lobe

Figure 3.2 This diagram shows the hypothalamus and pituitary glands. The pituitary is attached to the underside of the brain at the hypothalamus by a thin stalk. The anterior pituitary receives blood that contains controlling factors directly from the hypothalamus. These factors either stimulate or inhibit the release of pituitary hormones. The posterior pituitary is controlled by nerves from the hypothalamus.

The hypothalamus controls the **pituitary gland**, which is attached to the underside of the brain by a slender stalk. The pituitary gland, also called the **hypophysis** (hi-POF-ih-sis; Greek for "to grow under"), sits in a pocket of bone called the *sella turcica* ("Turk's saddle"), which is located directly above the palate of the mouth and behind the bridge of the nose. In the past, the pituitary has been called the "master gland" because it controls many other endocrine glands, but this term is no longer widely used. The word *pituitary* is derived from the

Latin *pituita,* or "phlegm," because early anatomists believed this gland produced saliva. The pituitary regulates the thyroid gland, adrenal glands, and the reproductive organs. It also produces hormones that control growth and kidney function, are involved in milk production, and are related to childbirth.

The pituitary gland has two parts: the anterior (adenohypophysis) and the posterior pituitary (neurohypophysis). During embryonic development, a fold of tissue moves up from the roof of the mouth and forms the anterior pituitary. A piece of the hypothalamus bulges downward to form the posterior portion. The two pieces of tissue join to create the pituitary gland. The anterior portion is physically separate from the brain, but is connected to it by a special type of blood circulation, called the **hypophyseal portal** or shunt. Capillaries in the hypothalamus join to form a vein that enters the pituitary gland and then separates to form capillaries. This system of circulation allows blood to pick up chemicals called "controlling factors" that are released in the hypothalamus and carry them directly to the pituitary gland, where they control the release of hormones. Every pituitary gland hormone has at least one releasing factor or hormone and some have both inhibiting and releasing factors.

The following hormones are released by the anterior pituitary:

- **Growth Hormone** stimulates bone and muscle cells to grow.

- **Prolactin** causes the mammary glands to produce milk.

- **Follicle Stimulating Hormone** (**FSH**) and **Luteinizing Hormone** (**LH**), known collectively as **gonadotropins**, stimulate hormone and gamete production by the **gonads** (testes and ovaries).

- **Thyroid Stimulating Hormone** (**TSH**) causes the thyroid to produce thyroid hormone.

- **Adrenocorticotropic Hormone** (**ACTH**) stimulates the adrenal cortex to produce corticosteroids, especially during periods of stress.

- **Melanocyte Stimulating Hormone** (**MSH**) may have a role in fat metabolism.

- **Endorphins**, which are also produced by the brain, reduce the perception of pain.

The posterior pituitary is an extension of the brain. It releases two hormones—**oxytocin** and **antidiuretic hormone** (ADH)—that are made in specialized cells in the hypothalamus. The hormones are transported down nerve cells into the pituitary, where they are stored. The hypothalamus signals for their release by direct nerve signals to allow for quicker secretion. Oxytocin stimulates the uterus to contract during labor and stimulates the breast to start releasing milk when a baby nurses. Antidiuretic hormone reduces urine output by acting on the collecting ducts of the kidney.

THE PINEAL GLAND

The **pineal gland**, a structure about the size of a pea, is located slightly above and behind the hypothalamus. The pineal gland receives information via the thalamus from the eyes about light and dark cycles. It is involved in rhythmic behavior, such as sleep cycles for humans, but it is much more complicated in animals. For example, the pineal gland is crucial in helping birds decide when it is time to fly south for the winter. The pineal gland secretes the hormone **melatonin**, a modified amino acid that is derived from the neurotransmitter serotonin. Melatonin is released at night and acts within the brain to affect the cyclic behaviors. During winter, the length of the dark period increases, so more melatonin is released. This release connects daily cycles with seasonal cycles. Humans, however, do not have seasonal behaviors like animals that only reproduce at certain times of the year. The significance of melatonin and the pineal gland in humans is not clear. Many people believe that the body produces less melatonin as it ages and that this is one of the causes of aging. Some people use over-the-counter preparations of melatonin to fight jetlag and insomnia because it helps adjust the body's sleep-wake cycle.

Scientists are fairly certain that melatonin levels are involved in **seasonal affective disorder** (**SAD**), a condition that can be debilitating. For some people, the reduced amount of daylight during winter produces a craving for carbohydrates and causes lethargy and sometimes depression. SAD is often treated by exposing the sufferer to elevated levels of full-spectrum light—light that has all of the wavelengths of sunlight (red to violet). Regular artificial lights do not have all of the wavelengths. Some individuals may be given melatonin and antidepressants as well.

THE THYROID GLAND
The thyroid gland is a butterfly-shaped structure located in front of the trachea (windpipe), between the larynx and the

SEASONAL AFFECTIVE DISORDER (SAD)
According to the National Mental Health Association, "SAD is a mood disorder associated with depression episodes and related to seasonal variations of light." This means that a person suffers from depression during the winter months, but the symptoms disappear in the spring. A diagnosis usually requires the symptoms to occur over three consecutive winters. SAD is more common in women than in men and usually begins between the ages of 18 and 30. The disorder occurs throughout the temporal regions of both the Northern and Southern hemispheres, but becomes more frequent—and more severe—as distance form the equator increases. This corresponds with the decreasing amount of daylight available during the winter months.

notch at the top of the rib cage. The thyroid gland secretes three hormones: **triiodothyronine** (T_3), **tetraiodothyronine** or **thyroxine** (T_4), and **calcitonin**. T_3 and T_4, which are collectively called "thyroid hormone," are very similar in structure and action. They are both derived from the amino acid **tyrosine**. T_3 has three iodine atoms, and T_4 has four. If a person's diet does not include sufficient iodine, the thyroid cannot produce enough thyroid hormone. The gland then enlarges, causing a visible swelling on the front of the neck. This is called a **goiter**. This disorder has been virtually eliminated by adding iodine to table salt.

Both T_3 and T_4 work in nearly all body tissues, but T_3 is more likely to attach to the target receptor, which is located in the nucleus of cells, where it can directly affect genes. The primary action of thyroid hormone is to increase metabolic rate. A person with low levels of thyroid hormone will tend to feel cold, be lethargic, and gain weight easily. Thyroid hormone also plays a critical role in development and growth. A baby with thyroid deficiency will have mental and growth retardation, a condition called **cretinism**. Chapter 5 will explain this condition in more detail.

Calcitonin lowers blood calcium levels by acting on bones and kidneys. Calcium is removed from the blood and stored in the bones. The kidneys reduce the amount of calcium that is returned to the blood and allow more to be excreted in the urine. This process is described in Chapter 8.

THE PARATHYROID GLANDS

The **parathyroid glands** are four small tissue masses attached to the back of the thyroid. They secrete parathyroid hormone (PTH), also called parathormone. PTH lowers blood calcium levels by stimulating its release from bone and stimulating its uptake by the kidneys and intestines. It has the opposite effect of the thyroid hormone calcitonin.

THE THYMUS GLAND

Although the **thymus** gland is technically part of the immune system, it also produces a chemical called **thymosin** that activates cells of the immune system called **lymphocytes**, or white blood cells. After lymphocytes have passed through the thymus or have come in contact with thymosin, they are referred to as T lymphocytes. These lymphocytes are involved in many aspects of immunity, including producing chemicals that stimulate and regulate the immune response. The thymus, located in the chest region, is prominent during infancy and childhood, but decreases in size as humans age.

THE PANCREAS

The pancreas, located beneath the stomach, is attached to the small intestine by the pancreatic duct through which digestive enzymes are released. The endocrine cells are scattered throughout the pancreas in little groups called **islets of Langerhans**. They were named in honor of Paul Langerhans, a German medical student who described them in 1869. The islets secrete two hormones, insulin and glucagon, which work to control blood glucose levels. Insulin is unique in that it is the only hormone that lowers blood glucose levels. Glucagon raises blood glucose levels, allowing us to maintain a nearly constant concentration of glucose in our blood in between meals. The homeostasis of blood glucose is described in Chapter 4.

THE ADRENAL GLANDS

The adrenal glands (Figure 3.3) sit above the kidneys (*ad* means "near" and *renal* means "kidney"). They are slightly triangular in shape and weigh about 4 g (0.14 ounces; about the same as a person's thumb). There are two distinct regions: the cortex, or outer layer, and the medulla, or inner region. During embryonic development, two separate cell populations migrate to the region near the kidneys and form the adrenal glands. One population is from nervous tissue and

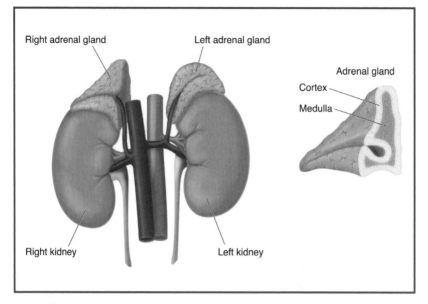

Figure 3.3 The adrenal glands, shown here, are small organs shaped almost like pyramids sitting on top of each kidney. Each gland has two layers. The outer layer, or cortex, secretes steroids like cortisone. The inner layer, or medulla, secretes epinephrine and norepinephrine.

forms the **adrenal medulla**, or middle. The outer layer of cells forms the **adrenal cortex**, which is controlled chemically by the anterior pituitary gland.

The adrenal medulla secretes epinephrine (adrenaline) and norepinephrine (noradrenaline). These hormones are released during periods of stress, causing the response known as fight-or-flight.

The adrenal gland secretes four groups of steroids, known as **corticosteroids: estrogens** (female sex hormones), **androgens** (male sex hormones), **glucocorticoids**, and **mineralocorticoids**. Released during times of stress, glucocorticoids raise blood glucose levels, decrease inflammation, and delay healing. Mineralocorticoids work on the kidneys to increase sodium and water reabsorption.

THE GONADS

The ovaries and the testes (the gonads) produce gametes and sex hormones. In females, the ovaries produce eggs and estrogens, the primary hormones that maintain the female reproductive tract and produce female secondary sexual characteristics. The ovaries also produce **progesterone**, the hormone released during pregnancy. Progesterone helps the uterus maintain the pregnancy. In males, the testes produce sperm and the androgens (male hormones). The primary male sex hormone is **testosterone**. The hormones of reproduction will be described in Chapter 6.

THE KIDNEYS

The two kidneys are located at the back of the abdominal cavity, just below the rib cage. The kidneys remove water-soluble wastes from the blood and regulate the osmotic balance of the body. They also help regulate blood pressure through the renin-angiotensin-aldosterone system and atrial natriuretic factor, which will be described in Chapter 8. When body tissues are exposed to low levels of oxygen, the kidneys convert a plasma protein to erythropoietin. This hormone stimulates the red bone marrow located in the ends of the long bones to produce more red blood cells (erythrocytes). Because red blood cells carry oxygen, this increases the amount of oxygen delivered to the tissues, which, in turn, causes the level of erythropoietin to be lowered so red blood cell production slows.

THE HEART

The human heart has four chambers. The two upper chambers, called the atria, receive the blood flowing into the heart. When the blood volume increases, cells in the atria release a protein called **atrial natriuretic factor** (ANF). This hormone causes blood vessels to dilate and the kidneys to produce more urine. The net result is to lower the blood pressure and reduce blood volume by excreting more water.

THE DIGESTIVE SYSTEM

The stomach and the small intestine secrete substances that control the digestive tract and appetite. The stomach begins to secrete gastric juices, which include hydrochloric acid, when food is present. It also secretes a hormone called gastrin into the blood, which stimulates the further secretion of gastric juices. As stomach acid is secreted, the pH in the stomach drops. When the pH reaches a certain level, the stomach does not secrete as much gastrin and, thus, the secretion of gastric juices also decreases. The stomach also produces a chemical called ghrelin that appears to be one of the signals to the brain that causes hunger.

The small intestine releases secretin when food enters from the stomach. This, in turn, stimulates the pancreas to release bicarbonate to neutralize the acid. If protein or fats are present in the food, cholecystokinin (CCK) is released. It stimulates the release of bile from the gallbladder and digestive enzymes from the pancreas. It also signals the brain that a person is "full." Another chemical called PYY3-36 also signals the brain to stop eating. Scientists believe that there are other chemicals involved in controlling digestion and whether or not a person feels hungry, some of which come from the digestive tract and some from other body parts, such as fat cells.

CONNECTIONS

The organs that secrete hormones are called endocrine glands. They are located throughout the body and may have other functions in addition to secreting hormones. Each endocrine gland secretes particular hormones that act on other parts of the body. These actions include regulating blood glucose concentrations, controlling reproduction, dealing with stress, maintaining body functions, and regulating ion concentrations. Table 3.1 summarizes the endocrine organs, their secretions, and their primary actions.

Table 3.1: Endocrine Organs and Their Actions

Gland	Hormone	Chemical Class of Hormone	Hormone Action
Hypothalamus	Releasing and inhibiting factors		Control anterior pituitary
Pituitary			
Anterior	Growth Hormone	Protein	Growth of bone and muscle
	Prolactin	Protein	Milk production
	FSH/LH	Protein	Gamete and hormone production
	Thyroid stimulating hormone (TSH)	Protein	Stimulates thyroid
	ACTH	Peptide	Stimulates adrenal cortex
Posterior	Oxytocin	Peptide	Uterine contractions
	ADH	Peptide	Reduce urine output
Pineal gland	Melatonin	Amine	Biological rhythms
Thyroid gland	T_3 & T_4	Amine	Stimulate metabolic rate
	Calcitonin	Peptide	Lower blood calcium
Parathyroid glands	Parathyroid hormone	Peptide	Raise blood calcium
Thymus	Thymosin	Peptide	Stimulates T lymphocytes
Pancreas	Insulin	Protein	Lower blood glucose
	Glucagon	Protein	Raise blood glucose
Adrenal glands			
Medulla	Epinephrine	Amine	Fight-or-flight
Cortex	Glucocorticoids	Steroid	Raise blood glucose
	Mineralocorticoids	Steroid	Absorb water and sodium in kidneys
Gonads			
Ovaries	Estrogens	Steroid	Female secondary sexual characteristics
	Progesterone	Steroid	Pregnancy
Testes	Androgens	Steroid	Male secondary sexual characteristics
Kidney	Erythropoietin	Peptide	Red blood cell production
	Renin	Peptide	Blood pressure and volume
Heart	Atrial natriuretic factor (ANF)	Peptide	Increase urine production, lower blood volume
Digestive system	Gastrin	Peptide	Secretion of gastric juices
	Secretin	Peptide	Pancreas releases HCO_3
	CCK	Peptide	Gallbladder releases bile; satiety (feeling full)

Table 3.1 Some endocrine glands secrete one hormone, while others secrete many. The primary hormones or class of hormones secreted by each gland are listed in this table, along with the chemical nature and primary action of each hormone, steroid, peptide, or amine.

4

Blood Glucose Levels

All living cells require energy to do work, such as producing new molecules, growing, and dividing. For most cells, the sugar molecule glucose ($C_6H_{12}O_6$) is the usual source of this energy. Glucose is provided by carbohydrates in the diet or by converting amino acids (the building blocks of protein) into glucose. Complex carbohydrates (starch) are digested into glucose molecules in the small intestine. The glucose molecules are transported into the blood and then delivered to all the cells of the body. The liver and muscle cells take in glucose and store it as a large molecule called glycogen that is similar to starch. Each glycogen molecule contains as many as one million glucose molecules. As much as 10% of the liver's weight can be made up of glycogen. When the body needs it, the liver breaks the glycogen apart to produce glucose through a process called **glycogenolysis** (*lysis* is Greek for "to loosen" or "split"). The glucose molecules are released into the bloodstream and shared with the entire body. Muscle cells also carry out glycogenolysis, but do not release the glucose. Glycogen formation is called **glycogenesis** (*genesis* comes from the Greek for "to be born").

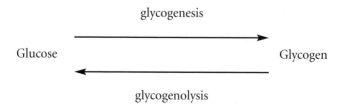

The amount of glucose in the blood is maintained at around 90 mg/100 ml of blood, but values between 70 and 105 mg/100 ml are considered normal for anyone between 2 and 50 years of age. (Note: Blood glucose levels are often reported in mg/dl, which is the same as mg/100 ml.) The blood glucose level is maintained primarily by two pancreatic hormones: glucagon and insulin. These two hormones have opposite reactions: Insulin lowers blood glucose, and glucagon raises it. Several other hormones also affect glucose levels, but not as directly or dramatically as glucagon and insulin do. Figure 4.1 shows the chemical structure of glucose and glycogen.

INSULIN AND GLUCAGON:
REGULATING GLUCOSE IN THE BLOOD
Insulin and glucagon, which are produced in the pancreas, are the primary hormones involved in regulating the level of glucose in the blood. The pancreas contains about one million isolated groups of cells called islets of Langerhans or pancreatic islets. The islets are about 1% of the pancreas by weight. There are two different kinds of islet cells: α (alpha) and β (beta) cells, which are involved in carbohydrate metabolism control. β cells secrete insulin, while α cells secrete glucagon.

Because proteins cannot pass through cell membranes, the receptors for insulin and glucagon must be on the cell membrane itself. When insulin and glucagon bind to protein receptors on the surface of the target cells, they initiate actions within the cell (recall Chapter 2). Insulin and glucagon affect carbohydrate, fat, and protein metabolism throughout the body, but the primary targets are liver, muscle, and adipose (fat) cells. Insulin is a unique hormone because it is the only one whose net effect is **hypoglycemic** (*hypo* comes from the Greek for "under" or "less")—that is, it lowers blood glucose levels. Glucagon has generally the opposite effect; it is **hyperglycemic** (*hyper* is Greek for "over" or "more").

After a person eats **carbohydrates** (sugars and starches), blood glucose levels rise. The β cells are stimulated directly by the glucose to release insulin into the blood. The insulin then

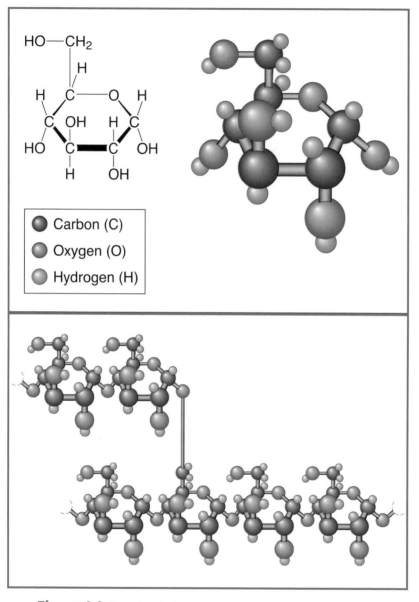

Figure 4.1 The chemical structure of glucose, $C_6H_{12}O_6$, is seen here (at top). Glucose is the energy source for most cells of the body. Glycogen is the storage form of glucose. It is a highly branched chain of about a million glucose molecules. The diagram at bottom shows just a tiny portion of a glycogen molecule.

travels throughout the body, enhancing the transport of glucose into cells, especially fat and muscle cells. Insulin affects fat cells by increasing the uptake and utilization of glucose. Fat synthesis then increases, and the hormones (growth hormone and epinephrine) that increase fat breakdown are opposed. Muscle cells also increase their uptake of glucose, which increases glycogen synthesis. Insulin also seems to increase amino acid transport and stimulate protein synthesis. Liver cells are stimulated to increase the incorporation of glucose into glycogen. This indirectly increases the transport of glucose into the cells, but increasing glucose transport is not a primary action of insulin on liver cells. Insulin also increases amino acid uptake and the subsequent protein synthesis by liver cells. In short, glucose stimulates the use of glucose, glycogenesis, **lipogenesis** (fat synthesis), and **proteogenesis** (protein synthesis). It opposes fat breakdown (**lipolysis**) and the formation of ketone bodies, which are the products of lipolysis. As the blood glucose level decreases, insulin secretion gradually decreases until the blood glucose level reaches about 80–85 mg of glucose/100 ml of blood.

In contrast, when the blood glucose level reaches about 50 mg/100 ml, the α-islet cells begin to secrete glucagon. Glucagon stimulates the liver cells to begin glycogenolysis, quickly raising blood glucose levels. Proteins in the liver and muscle cells are broken down into amino acids that are released into the bloodstream and sent to the liver. Their conversion to glucose (**gluconeogenesis**) is stimulated in the liver by glucagon. Liver and fat cells begin to mobilize and break down fat molecules. Potassium levels in the blood also rise, probably as a side effect of the glycogenolysis. Glucagon also stimulates the β cells directly, causing them to release insulin, which may increase the body cells' ability to utilize the newly released glucose. Animals that are given injections of pure glucagon fail to gain weight, reduce their food consumption, and break down body proteins. The activity of their digestive tracts also decreases.

The net effect of these two hormones is to keep blood glucose levels within very narrow limits. When blood glucose level increases, insulin release is stimulated, and glucagon release is inhibited. Glucose leaves the blood and is utilized by cells, especially liver, fat, and muscle cells. When blood glucose level decreases, glucagon is secreted, causing glucose to be released from its storage form, glycogen, in the liver, thus raising blood glucose levels. Both hormones are released simultaneously when someone eats a diet high in protein and low in carbohydrates, apparently because certain amino acids are present that have a stimulatory action on both hormones. Glucagon counteracts insulin's stimulation of fat synthesis. This counteractive action, in part, accounts for the rapid weight loss that can occur with high-protein diets. Figure 4.2 shows how these two hormones work together to maintain blood glucose homeostasis.

ADRENAL HORMONES

The adrenal glands secrete epinephrine and norepinephrine. The glands secrete epinephrine when a person feels stressed, either physically because of an injury or psychologically. One effect of the release of epinephrine is a rapid rise in blood glucose, which provides an energy source for cells. This happens in two ways. First, epinephrine blocks insulin release and stimulates glucagon release. Second, epinephrine acts directly on liver cells to stimulate glycogenolysis. It also causes fat cells to release fatty acids (components of fat). Both of these responses provide cells with more fuel, so the body can better deal with the stress.

During longer periods of stress (hours to days), the adrenal cortex releases glucocorticoids, such as cortisol. These hormones inhibit protein synthesis and stimulate protein breakdown. The resulting amino acids can be converted to glucose in the liver, thus raising blood levels.

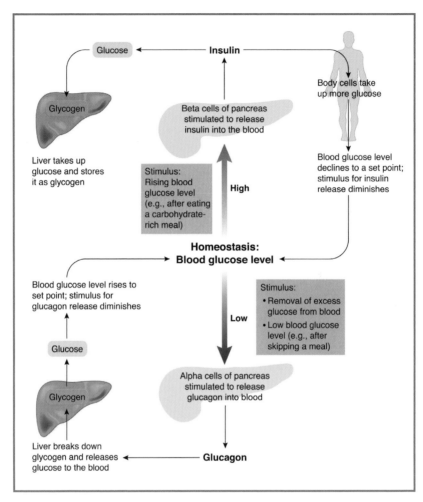

Figure 4.2 Glucose homeostasis helps regulate blood sugar levels. Blood glucose levels are maintained primarily by the antagonistic actions of insulin and glucagon. Both hormones are secreted from the pancreas in response to the amount of glucose in the blood. Insulin lowers glucose levels, whereas glucagon raises them.

OTHER HORMONES AND CHEMICALS

Growth hormone and thyroid hormone affect metabolism, so they have some indirect effects on blood glucose levels. Growth hormone raises blood glucose levels and also reduces the sensitivity of the cell membrane receptors to insulin. Thyroid hormone can cause hypoglycemia by increasing the rate at which cells use glucose.

Many drugs and chemicals can affect blood glucose levels. Some act by directly opposing the action of insulin or glucagon. Others enhance or inhibit hormone release, destroy or protect the hormone, or affect the membrane receptors. Among the drugs known to affect glucose levels are the sulfa drugs (antibiotics); diuretics such as thiazide; oral contraceptives; phenytoin (Dilantin®), which is used to treat epilepsy; cyclosporine (an immune suppressant given to transplant patients); and opiates, such as morphine.

DIABETES MELLITUS

The American Diabetes Association estimates that almost 16 million Americans have diabetes. In 2000, approximately 69,000 deaths in the United States were attributed to diabetes. It is ranked as the sixth leading cause of death in the United States.

Diabetes is not one disease but a group of metabolic disorders characterized primarily by elevated blood glucose levels. The most common form (found in about 90% of diabetic Americans) is **non-insulin-dependent diabetes mellitus** (NIDDM), also called **type 2** or **age-onset diabetes**. This form can be caused by decreased or irregular release of insulin or, most commonly, by reduced sensitivity of the receptors to insulin. Obesity drastically increases the risk of developing NIDDM. The onset is usually gradual and is often not recognized. Severity of the disease is determined by the amount of glucose in the blood. If the levels are less than 126 mg/100 ml, treatment will usually be as simple as increasing exercise and controlling the diet. Most people with NIDDM are older than 40 and are obese.

The second most common form of diabetes (about 10% of diabetics) is **insulin-dependent diabetes mellitus** (IDDM), also called **type 1** or **juvenile-onset diabetes**. This form begins earlier in life and is caused by the destruction of islet cells by the victim's own immune system over a period of years. One of the serious acute symptoms of IDDM is the accumulation of chemicals called ketones in the blood. These chemicals (e.g., acetone) lower the blood pH, producing a condition called **ketoacidosis**. This condition can cause coma and even death if untreated. Before Banting and Best isolated insulin, most type 1 diabetics died within a year of being diagnosed. Insulin from animals (pigs and horses) was used to treat diabetics until recombinant DNA technology made the production of human insulin possible. Insulin injections prolong the life of the diabetic and reduce symptoms, but they do not cure the disease. There currently is no cure, although transplantation of pancreas tissue is regarded as one possible option.

DIABETES AND BIRTH DEFECTS

Women who have diabetes when they become pregnant are 2–5 times more likely to have a baby with a serious congenital malformation (a body part that has not formed correctly). One of the most common is a neural tube defect that affects the brain and/or spinal cord. Based on research done on diabetic mice, it appears that elevated glucose levels may influence the expression of genes that control cell development.

Human organ formation occurs during the embryonic period that lasts from conception to the eighth week of development. The brain and spinal cord are the first organs to form. The critical time for preventing neural tube defects actually occurs even before the mother has missed her first period— before she even knows she is pregnant. Diabetic women who are contemplating getting pregnant must tightly control their blood glucose before conception occurs. According to the American Diabetic Association, women who monitored their blood glucose level "lowered their baby's risk of birth defects to only 1%, compared with 10% in babies of mothers who began intensive diabetes management after conceiving."

Gestational diabetes (GDM), which is similar to NIDDM, can occur when a woman is pregnant and usually disappears as soon as she gives birth. An elevated blood glucose level in the mother is rarely life-threatening to the fetus, but it is related to increased complications during pregnancy and birth. Gestational diabetes is also an indicator of an increased risk of developing type 2 diabetes later in life. Treatment includes diet management and insulin injections.

The elevated blood glucose level, excess fatty acids in the blood, and insulin resistance found in diabetes patients cause damage to the cells that line the blood vessels of the eyes, kidneys, extremities, and the heart. This damage is part of the reason that diabetics are at high risk for blindness, kidney failure, amputations, stroke, and heart attack. According to an epidemiological study published in the *Journal of the American Medical Association* in May 2002, most patients with diabetes die from complications of atherosclerosis (the buildup of fatty plaques inside arteries).

The actual causes of all types of diabetes are not known. What is known at this time is that genetics plays a large role in all forms of the disease. Both type 1 and type 2 diabetes seem to be hereditary. Caucasians are more likely to get type 1 diabetes than are other racial groups, but people of African, Native American, Asian, and Hispanic (excluding Cuban) descent are more likely to develop type 2 diabetes. A number of genes have been identified that make a person more likely to develop type 1 diabetes, but there does not appear to be a specific "diabetes gene." Age, a sedentary lifestyle, and obesity are associated with increased risk of type 2 diabetes. Obesity is defined as being more than 120% of a person's ideal body weight. In addition, the location of the body fat seems to be important in determining risk. Having fat located above the hips (in the central body cavity) increases a person's risk more than having fat on the hips.

Millions of Americans are living with diabetes. This means that the disease can be controlled. Elevated blood glucose levels can affect nearly every aspect of a person's life as well as his or her body. Often, the help of a number of individuals in addition to a physician is required. For example, the American Diabetes Association suggests that a diabetic patient consult a registered dietitian at least once a year. Eating habits and other behaviors that have developed over a lifetime may have to be changed, sometimes dramatically. Diabetics often have problems with their eyes and extremities (hands, feet, and legs) due to cell damage and poor blood circulation. Help with exercise, eye and foot care, as well as education, can contribute significantly to the long-term health of a diabetic.

CONNECTIONS

Human cells need a constant supply of fuel. Most of the body's cells preferentially use glucose as their energy source. Glucose is supplied to cells via the blood. The concentration of glucose in the blood plasma must be maintained at high enough levels to supply the cells adequately, but not high enough to cause tissue damage. The delicate balance of glucose homeostasis is maintained by the counterbalancing effects of glucagon and insulin. Glucose is removed from the blood and utilized by cells or stored in liver and muscle cells as the polymer glycogen when insulin is present. Liver glycogen can be converted back to glucose and amino acids can be converted into glucose by liver cells when insulin is absent and glucagon is present, thus increasing blood glucose levels. The hormone epinephrine also stimulates glycogenolysis. Blood glucose level can change according to diet, external stimuli, or taking drugs or ingesting other substances.

5

Growth and Metabolism

How tall a human being will be as an adult depends on many factors. First and foremost is genetics; tall parents tend to have tall children and short parents tend to have short children. In addition to genes, several hormones affect growth and development either directly or indirectly. The two most important hormones are growth hormone (GH) and thyroid hormone. The sex hormones, testosterone and estrogen, have significant impacts on the timing of growth. Testosterone and estrogen also affect the metabolic rate, which can be described as how the body uses its energy sources. In this chapter, each hormone and some of the common growth and metabolic disorders associated with them will be examined.

GROWTH HORMONE

Growth hormone (GH), also called **somatotrophin**, is secreted by the anterior pituitary gland under the control of two hormones from the hypothalamus. Growth hormone releasing hormone (GHRH) stimulates the pituitary to release GH. When GH levels are high enough, feedback to the hypothalamus inhibits GHRH and stimulates instead the release of **somatostatin**, the second factor from the hypothalamus, which slows GH release. Somatostatin also inhibits other pituitary hormones, digestive tract hormones, and all pancreatic secretions.

Growth hormone can be considered an **anabolic** hormone, meaning it stimulates synthesis—specifically, protein synthesis in bone and muscle. It stimulates the use of fat as fuel so that lean body mass increases and the skeleton grows. Growth hormone has direct and indirect effects throughout the body. Fat and liver tissues are affected directly to release fat molecules, decrease glucose uptake, and increase glycogenolysis (breakdown of glycogen to glucose). The indirect effects are more widespread. GH stimulates liver, kidney, muscle, bone, and cartilage cells to release proteins called insulin-like growth factors (IGFs). These molecules increase protein synthesis, cell division, and growth, and, in particular, stimulate cartilage growth. This leads to skeletal growth. Humans gain height as long as the bones continue to lengthen. Bones grow at their ends, at areas called growth plates. Once the growth plates in the bones are sealed, the person cannot grow any taller, but soft tissues can always continue to grow and respond to GH.

GROWTH HORMONE DISORDERS

Growth hormone deficiency (GHD) will cause abnormally short stature called pituitary **dwarfism**. People with this disorder will usually have normally proportioned bodies, but only reach a height of about 4 feet. Babies born with this disorder are normal in length at birth, but usually have some type of medical problem, such as low blood sugar or jaundice, which warrants further testing. In the past, the only way to treat dwarfism was to extract pituitaries from cadavers to supply GH. Unfortunately, because GH is produced in minute quantities in the pituitary gland and degrades quickly, this treatment did not produce enough of the hormone to treat all the children who needed it. With the advent of recombinant DNA technology, it became possible to produce human growth hormone in greater quantities. It is now possible for affected children to receive injections of growth hormone and to achieve normal heights. The biggest disadvantage is that GH therapy is still very expensive, costing up to $20,000 a year.

If too much GH is produced before the bones stop growing, the person will be taller than normal, at 7–8 feet tall. This condition is called **gigantism**. If excess GH is released when the person is already an adult, the person suffers from **acromegaly**.

A person with this condition displays several characteristics. Because the bones cannot elongate, they tend to widen, especially in the hands and feet. Soft tissues (like the layers between the skin and muscles) thicken. The nose becomes wide, the ears and chin grow, and the tongue enlarges.

It is difficult to directly measure GH levels because GH is not released continuously. Growth hormone is secreted primarily at night while we are sleeping. For this reason, if excess GH secretion is suspected, doctors will measure it indirectly by measuring IGF (insulin-like growth factors) levels.

THYROID HORMONE

Growth hormone and thyroid hormone (TH) are **synergists**, which means they increase each other's effectiveness to promote normal growth and development. Neither hormone alone can cause normal growth. For example, if there is not enough TH present during gestation or infancy, the baby will have a form of growth and mental retardation called cretinism, even if GH levels are normal. These children will be very short, have pot-bellies, and have a protruding tongue and mental retardation.

The release of thyroid hormone is controlled by the hypothalamus and pituitary via a classic feedback mechanism. When TH levels decrease, the hypothalamus releases thyroid stimulating hormone releasing factor (TSH-RF), which, in turn, signals the pituitary to release thyroid stimulating hormone. The release of TSH causes the thyroid to synthesize and release more TH. The rising TH levels in the blood tell the hypothalamus to stop secreting TSH-RF. The pituitary stops secreting TSH and, consequently, the thyroid slows the release of TH. It appears that TH may also act on the pituitary to inhibit TSH release directly. This is shown in Figure 5.1.

Thyroid hormone is actually a mixture of two hormones: triiodothyronine (T_3) and tetraiodothyronine (T_4 or thyroxine). Both of these are synthesized from the amino acid tyrosine in a multistep process in the thyroid. The major chemical difference

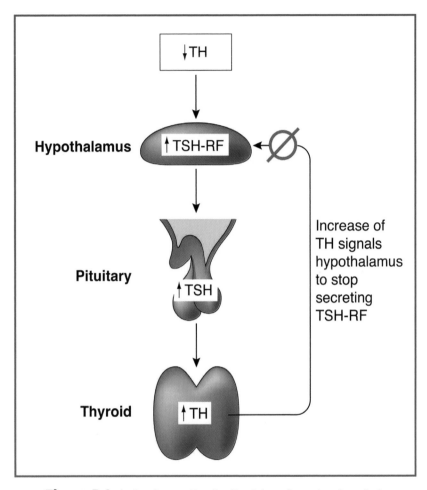

Figure 5.1 A classic negative feedback loop (seen here) controls the release of thyroid hormone. When thyroid hormone (TH) levels fall, the hypothalamus sends thyroid stimulating hormone releasing factor (TSH-RF) to the pituitary, which then releases thyroid stimulating hormone (TSH). TSH causes the thyroid to secrete more TH. As TH levels increase, the hypothalamus stops secreting TSH-RF.

between the two is that T_3 has three iodine atoms and T_4 has four. In several tissues of the body, especially the kidney, T_4 is changed into T_3. T_3 is faster and more effective than T_4 at producing its metabolic activities.

Besides being necessary for normal growth and development, TH also stimulates the metabolism of nearly every tissue of the body. It controls **basal metabolic rate** (BMR), or how much energy, measured in kilocalories, the body needs just to keep itself going. T_3 is small enough to enter the cell through the cell membrane. It attaches to receptor proteins in the nucleus and turns on genes, so that certain enzymes are produced. The net effect on nearly every organ is that oxygen consumption increases and more energy is used. When cells produce energy, they generate heat, so the body becomes warmer and thus more tolerant of cold conditions. To provide more glucose, the main source of this cellular energy, T_3 also stimulates glucose absorption in the intestine and glycogenolysis and gluconeogenesis in the liver (recall Chapter 4). Normal levels of TH stimulate protein synthesis and the mobilization of fat stores.

HYPOTHYROIDISM

As mentioned earlier, if TH levels are low during gestation or infancy, the baby will have retarded growth and mental development. **Hypothyroidism** in both mother and child is often caused by iodine deficiency because the thyroid needs iodine to make TH. The World Health Organization (WHO) estimates that "nearly 50 million people suffer from some degree of iodine deficiency disorder-related brain damage." Infants are screened for thyroid activity because low TH levels are one cause of mental retardation that is treatable. If inadequate iodine is the problem, simply adding a small amount to the diet will eliminate the problem. Otherwise, thyroid hormone can be given directly. This is called "replacement therapy," because the natural source is being replaced by an outside source of the hormone. If not treated, the child will be permanently retarded. Later in childhood, lack of TH will have less effect on mental ability, but will still impede normal growth. The child will appear to be younger than he or she actually is. Sexual development will also be delayed.

Hypothyroidism in adults usually develops slowly. It may begin with nonspecific symptoms such as feeling tired, lethargic, and experiencing constipation. Impaired mental and motor functions, such as slow reflexes, decreased appetite, and feeling cold are classic manifestations of insufficient thyroid hormone. In women, the menstrual flow is often heavier than normal. Infertility may occur. Changes in the skin are also typical. The skin feels dry, the nails are brittle, and hair loss occurs. Substances called **mucopolysaccharides**, large molecules made of protein and sugar, accumulate in the skin and organs. This accumulation causes the face to look round and puffy and the hands and feet to swell, a condition called myxedema. With longstanding hypothyroidism, **hypothermia**, or low body temperature, and even coma are possible.

HYPERTHYROIDISM

When more TH is secreted, the basal metabolic rate (BMR) is elevated so more energy is used, thus producing more heat. A person with **hyperthyroidism** typically feels warmer than normal and may also appear nervous and irritable due to increased sensitivity in the nervous system. The person often loses weight, but because the appetite also increases, these effects may offset each other. Bowel movements become more frequent, and heart rate increases. In fact, the person may feel like his or her heart is racing, even during sleep.

Graves' disease is the most common cause of hyperthyroidism. It is an autoimmune disorder in which the body's own immune system attacks and attaches to the TSH receptors in the thyroid, causing excess TH to be released. Most people with Graves' disease have an enlarged thyroid called a goiter. In addition, their eyes seem to bulge out because mucopolysaccharides have accumulated in the eye socket (Figure 5.2). If enough mucopolysaccharides build up in the eye socket, it may cause paralysis of the eye or double vision.

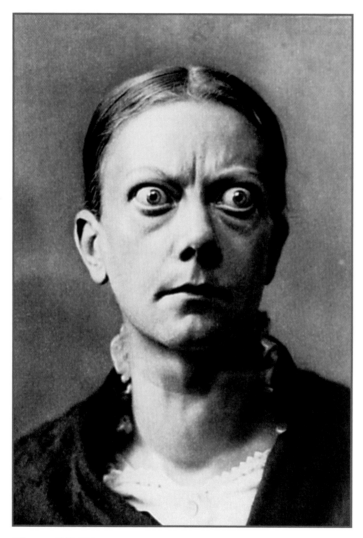

Figure 5.2 This woman shows the classic symptoms of an overactive thyroid, called hyperthyroidism. Usually this is caused by Graves' disease. The enlarged thyroid, seen on her neck, is called goiter. Her eyes seem to protrude, because of a buildup of tissue in the eye socket.

TREATMENT OF THYROID DISORDERS

Hypothyroidism due to iodine deficiency has been virtually eliminated in the United States and much of the world by adding iodine to table salt. Hypothyroidism caused by other factors is treated by replacing the missing TH. This treatment was first reported in 1891 by George R. Murray (1865–1939) in Great Britain. He injected a "glycerin extract of sheep's thyroid" under the skin to treat his patients. Today, patients are given synthetic human thyroxine, which is quickly converted to active T_3 in the body.

The treatment for hyperthyroidism varies according to the cause. If tumors in the thyroid are the root cause of the excess secretion or if the person cannot be treated with chemicals because of allergy or pregnancy, for example, part of the thyroid gland may be surgically removed. Since the 1940s, radioactive iodine has been available to treat hyperthyroidism. Because the thyroid gland is the only organ that uses iodine, the radioactive iodine only goes to that gland, where it accumulates within the cells and destroys some of them. The levels of radioactivity are very low and will disappear very quickly, so there is very little risk to the person being treated or to those around him or her. There are also drugs available that will alleviate some of the symptoms of an overactive thyroid. Because these drugs do not actually cure the disease, they are often used in conjunction with radioactive iodine or surgery until the levels of TH are normalized. Some drugs are now being developed that will inhibit the release or the activity of TH at the receptor level. Table 5.1 compares normal TH effects, hypothyroidism, and hyperthyroidism.

OTHER GROWTH REGULATORS

Testosterone, the male sex hormone, and estrogen, the female sex hormone, both affect growth. They both tend to accelerate growth, especially during the puberty growth spurt. Although girls usually begin their growth period earlier than boys do, estrogen tends to cause the growth plates of the bones to close so that girls stop growing before boys do. Because testosterone causes protein synthesis, especially in muscles, some athletes

Table 5.1 Effects of Thyroid Hormone

	Normal Levels of Thyroid Hormone	Hypothyroidism	Hyperthyroidism
Basal Metabolic Rate	Promotes normal use of oxygen and calories.	Lowered BMR and body temperature, fatigue, weight gain.	Increased BMR and body temperature, weight loss.
Food Metabolism	Increases glucose breakdown, fat usage, protein and cholesterol synthesis.	Protein synthesis and glucose usage decrease, blood cholesterol levels rise, fluid retention.	Breakdown of glucose, protein, and fat; loss of muscle mass.
Nervous System	Is necessary for normal development of fetus and child, and for normal function in adult.	Permanent retardation in infants. Slowed reflexes, loss of mental acuity in adults.	Increased sensitivity to adrenaline; nervousness and irritability.
Circulatory System	Promotes normal heart functions.	Lowered heart rate and blood pressure, decreased efficiency.	Increased heart rate and blood pressure.
Bones and Muscles	Is necessary for normal growth and development.	Short stature with disproportionate body; slower muscle movement, especially in digestive tract; arthritis.	Both become weaker in adults, calcium loss from bones, protein loss from muscles, speeds up movement in digestive tract.
Reproduction	Is necessary for normal female reproduction.	Heavier menstrual flow; egg production impaired, producing infertility; reduced milk production.	Lighter menstrual flow, possible infertility, impotence in males.
Hair and Skin	Regulates normal oil and sweat secretion.	Dry thick skin and coarse hair, brittle nails, loss of hair, face puffy.	Hair fine and soft, hair loss, nails soft, increased sweating.
Thyroid Gland	Controls normal size and shape of gland.	Goiter: thyroid gland swells while trying to synthesize more TH.	Enlarged due to hyperactivity.

Table 5.1 Thyroid hormone (TH) affects nearly every system in the body. The second column summarizes the effects of normal TH levels. The third describes what happens when levels of TH are too low, and the fourth describes the results of too much TH.

take various forms of testosterone, called anabolic steroids, to enhance muscle development.

Glucocorticoids, such as cortisol, are released from the adrenal cortex under the control of ACTH (adrenal corticotropic

ANABOLIC STEROIDS

Testosterone is the naturally occurring male sex hormone and, thus, it stimulates protein synthesis. This is one reason why males tend to be larger than females. Chemically, all the sex hormones, male and female, are steroids (see Chapter 2). Any chemical that is like testosterone and can stimulate protein synthesis is called an anabolic steroid. *Anabolic* means to "grow tissue." Some athletes inject or swallow synthetic and natural forms of these chemicals to enhance their muscle-building efforts. Steroids are not available without a prescription in the United States. They are, however, available in other countries, from some veterinarians, or they can be diverted from legal sources or produced in illegal laboratories.

There are both physical and psychological risks to using anabolic steroids, including an increased risk of liver, kidney, and prostate cancer. In addition, these steroids cause blood pressure and blood cholesterol levels to rise, so there is an increased risk of heart attack and stroke. Although many synthetic steroid products stimulate protein creation, they cannot signal the testes to produce sperm—a function that is controlled only by natural testosterone. As a result, many men who take these products experience decreased sperm production and shrunken testicles. In humans, if sperm production is reduced by only 50%, a man becomes functionally sterile. Many areas of the brain have receptors for testosterone. This means that steroid users may experience emotional changes such as mood swings, aggressive behavior, and even psychotic rages, depression, and delusions.

In young males, steroid use can cause bone growth to stop early, so users end up shorter than they would have been had they not used steroids. In females, the menstrual cycle becomes irregular, and facial hair and increased body hair may appear. Testosterone stimulates the oil and sweat glands, so individuals who take it often get acne. Male pattern baldness is inherited, but the gene is only expressed in the presence of testosterone. By artificially elevating testosterone levels, users also risk going bald. Figure 5.3 summarizes the effects of anabolic steroids.

Some substances that can be converted into testosterone or testosterone-like compounds are sold legally in the United States. These include DHEA (dehydroepian-drosterone) and androstene-dione (andro). They are sold, tested, and regulated as dietary supplements even though they are not food products, but synthetics. Little is known about their short- or long-term effects.

Many agencies and athletic groups are working to reduce the use of steroids by athletes, especially young athletes. A few of them are listed in the Appendix.

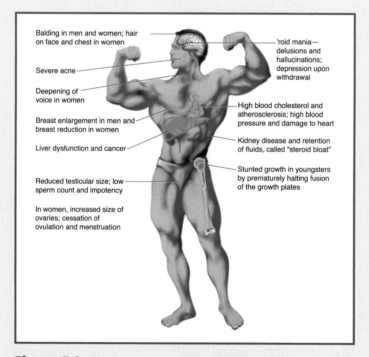

Balding in men and women; hair on face and chest in women

Severe acne

Deepening of voice in women

Breast enlargement in men and breast reduction in women

Liver dysfunction and cancer

Reduced testicular size; low sperm count and impotency

In women, increased size of ovaries; cessation of ovulation and menstruation

'roid mania—delusions and hallucinations; depression upon withdrawal

High blood cholesterol and atherosclerosis; high blood pressure and damage to heart

Kidney disease and retention of fluids, called "steroid bloat"

Stunted growth in youngsters by prematurely halting fusion of the growth plates

Figure 5.3 Anabolic steroids have a negative impact on many body functions. Because they are similar to testosterone, they affect reproduction and can cause sterility. Many of these effects are permanent and some can even be lethal.

hormone) from the hypothalamus. Excess glucocorticoids interfere with normal growth by increasing a person's weight but not height. In addition, cartilage and bone formation are directly impeded, muscles become weaker, and the person bruises easily, due at least partially to protein loss. Both testosterone and glucocorticoids raise blood glucose levels and increase lipolysis, but cortisol actually decreases the use of glucose by cells.

CONNECTIONS

Growth, development, and metabolism depend on a number of factors, both internal (such as genetics) and external (such as nutrition). Both growth hormone and thyroid hormone work together to promote normal growth and development and are essential for maintaining adult functional capabilities. Growth hormone from the pituitary gland is primarily responsible for growth after birth. In adults, it helps maintain muscle mass and mental faculties. TH is essential during pregnancy and throughout childhood for normal mental development as well as physical growth. TH maintains a normal metabolic rate and mental acuity. Too much or too little of either hormone can have profound effects on the body as well.

The sex hormones help determine the timing and duration of the growth spurt that occurs during puberty. Glucocorticoids increase the amount of glucose available to cells, but excess amounts will seriously impair skeletal growth and strength.

6

Reproduction

Hormones are involved in every aspect of reproduction. During development, hormones determine the sexual physical characteristics and produce and maintain the physical traits that are associated with being "male" and "female." Estrogens produce female characteristics, and testosterone produces male characteristics. Hormones control the production of gametes, eggs, and sperm, and control pregnancy, birth, milk production, and nursing.

EMBRYONIC DEVELOPMENT

Humans begin as a fertilized egg called a zygote. Shortly after fertilization, cell division begins. During the next 8–10 weeks, the embryonic period of development, the embryo enters the uterus and attaches to the wall. The extra embryonic membranes (the amnion and placenta) form. The amnion is the fluid-filled bag that completely surrounds the developing embryo. The placenta is a spongy disk-shaped structure that attaches to the uterine wall. The embryo is attached to the placenta by the umbilical cord. At the placenta, maternal and embryonic blood is separated by only a few cells. Substances such as oxygen and glucose diffuse from mother to embryo, and wastes diffuse in the opposite direction.

During the embryonic period, all the organs, including the organs of reproduction, develop. A female embryo will produce estrogens that cause the brain to develop into a female pattern brain to produce a monthly cycle. The female reproductive tract (ovaries, uterus, and vagina) and mammary glands develop. A male embryo produces testosterone and develops testes. The testosterone causes a male pattern brain to develop and causes male reproductive and urinary tracts to form.

If no testosterone is produced during the embryonic period, the embryo will develop into a functional female even though it is genetically male. It is presumed that this abnormal development occurs because of the large amount of estrogens present in the mother's body during pregnancy.

MALE REPRODUCTION

At puberty, the male hypothalamus begins to produce **gonadotropin releasing hormone (GnRH)**. This hormone is a small peptide that acts on the pituitary and stimulates it to release two proteins called luteinizing hormone (LH) and follicle stimulating hormone (FSH). Together, LH and FSH are called gonadotropins because they stimulate the gonads. These two hormones are also found in females; in fact, they are named for their actions in females.

Both FSH and LH act on the testes. FSH causes sperm production, while LH causes testosterone production. Testosterone inhibits the release of GnRH by the hypothalamus and gonadotropin release by the pituitary. As puberty progresses, the amount of testosterone required to inhibit the hypothalamus increases until about age 17, when the threshold is established. After this age, testosterone and sperm production will remain fairly constant throughout a male's adult life unless environmental or health factors intervene.

During puberty, testosterone stimulates the development of male secondary sexual characteristics, the physical features associated with being male. The voice deepens, facial hair appears, and skeletal and muscle growth is stimulated. In addition, sperm production begins. Growth in height and muscle mass begins during early puberty when it is usually most rapid, and continues for several years, often until age 21 and occasionally until age 25. Figure 6.1 shows how male growth hormones are released.

FEMALE REPRODUCTION

The female gonad, the ovary, produces the eggs and two types of steroid hormones: estrogens and progestins. Estrogens refer to several female sex hormones, including estradiol, estrone, and estriol. Technically, there is no one chemical called "estrogen." Whenever the term *estrogen* is used, it may be referring to all female sex hormones in a generic manner, to a mixture of hormones, or to just one of the hormones, depending on the context. Progesterone is the primary progestin secreted by the ovary.

Puberty usually begins around age 11 in girls, but it may occur as early as age 8. In females, the hypothalamus begins to produce gonadotropin releasing hormone (GnRH) just as in the male, but with one significant difference. The female hypothalamus releases GnRH cyclically, not continuously. At the onset of puberty, the amount of both gonadotropins (FSH and LH) released by the pituitary increases, but especially the amount of LH. This increase, in turn, stimulates the ovary to produce estradiol, which causes the development of female secondary sexual characteristics. These characteristics include breast development, maturation of the reproductive organs, and deposition of fat under the skin, especially on the hips and breasts. The pelvis widens, causing the hip socket to rotate forward and out. Estrogens also tend to cause the connective tissue of the musculoskeletal system (cartilage, tendons, and ligaments) to relax. This change means that teenage female athletes may be more prone to tendon and ligament injuries than males are.

The first menstrual period (menarche) occurs around the age of 12. Under the influence of estrogens, the uterine lining (endometrium) increases in thickness. When estrogen levels fall, the lining is sloughed off, producing the menstrual flow.

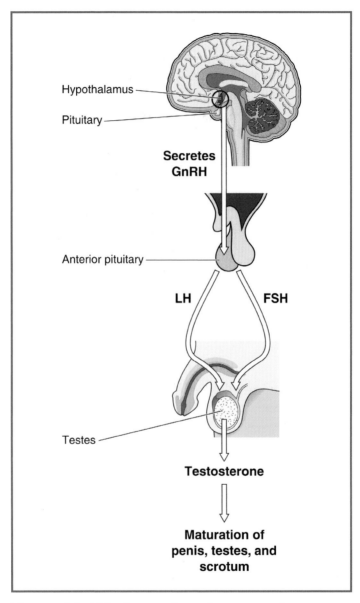

Hypothalamus

Pituitary

Secretes GnRH

Anterior pituitary

LH   **FSH**

Testes

Testosterone

Maturation of penis, testes, and scrotum

Figure 6.1 This diagram shows the process of testosterone production. The hypothalamus in the brain secretes gonadotropin releasing hormone (GnRH). GnRH then stimulates the pituitary to release the gonadotropins, LH and FSH. These two hormones stimulate the testes to produce testosterone and sperm.

The first ovulation (release of an egg from the ovary) will usually occur 6–9 months after menarche.

THE MENSTRUAL CYCLE

The female reproductive cycle normally lasts about 25–35 days. During this time, an egg will mature and be released from the ovary (a process called ovulation), ready to be fertilized. The uterus will be prepared to receive and accept a pregnancy. Once ovulation has occurred, the ovary will secrete hormones to maintain pregnancy. If fertilization does not occur, the egg disintegrates, the uterine lining is shed, and the process begins again with the next cycle.

The menstrual cycle starts when the hypothalamus secretes GnRH, stimulating the pituitary to release FSH and LH. The gonadotropins act on the ovary, which increases estrogen production. The estrogens slow gonadotropin release, but stimulate its synthesis and storage in the pituitary. At the same time, FSH makes one follicle, a group of cells that contain the eggs in the ovary, mature.

Estrogen levels continue to increase until they reach a critical level at about day 12 or 13 in the cycle. A burst of LH and a small amount of FSH are released, causing ovulation at mid-cycle (approximately day 14 of a 28-day cycle). At about the same time, chemicals called prostaglandins are released. Because these prostaglandins are phospholipids that are involved in many body responses, including the inflammatory response, the body temperature rises slightly at the time of ovulation. Once the egg has been released from the ovary, estrogen levels decrease, probably because the follicle was the primary source of the hormone. LH stimulates the ruptured follicle to become a structure called the corpus luteum, which begins to secrete progesterone (the hormone of pregnancy) and estrogen.

As progesterone and estrogen levels rise, they exert negative feedback on the hypothalamus and pituitary to decrease FSH and LH release. The egg enters the fallopian tube, where fertilization takes place. If fertilization does not occur, the corpus luteum degenerates, and estrogen and progesterone levels fall drastically, allowing FSH and LH secretion to increase again, and the cycle repeats.

Meanwhile, the uterus also responds to the hormonal

HORMONES AND BIRTH CONTROL

The most widely used form of birth control in the United States is the oral contraceptive, or birth control pill. Usually, these pills are given in 28-day packs. The first 21 pills, taken during the first 21 days of the woman's cycle, contain a combination of small doses of estrogens and progestins (synthetic progesterone). The levels of hormone contained in each pill are just high enough to mimic the effects of pregnancy on the hypothalamus, so GnRH is not released. The pituitary does not produce gonadotropins, so follicles do not mature; therefore, ovulation does not occur. The last seven pills of the cycle do not contain any hormones, so the levels of estrogen and progestin decrease. The endometrium (uterine lining), which has thickened, is sloughed off as menstrual flow.

If large doses of estrogen-progesterone combination pills are taken within 72 hours after having sexual intercourse, the menstrual cycle can be sufficiently interrupted to prevent fertilization or implantation of a fertilized egg. These pills are available in hospital emergency rooms for rape victims. They are widely used in Europe and Canada and are now available by prescription in the United States.

Mifepristone (RU-486) has been used for many years in Europe. This chemical blocks the receptors for progesterone in the uterus. When given with a small dose of prostaglandins during the first seven weeks of pregnancy, the uterus begins to contract and the embryo is expelled. The result is a chemically induced abortion. The drug is not used in the United States because of ethical and safety concerns.

changes. At the start of the menstrual cycle, estrogen and progesterone levels are low. The uterine lining (called the endometrium) detaches from the wall, causing blood and the uterine lining to pass out through the vagina for about 5 days. FSH and LH levels rise, stimulating estrogen to be secreted from the follicle. The endometrium becomes thick and full of blood vessels. Progesterone receptors develop and the mucus of the cervix becomes thin and develops channels to ease the movement of sperm. The uterus is almost ready to accept a pregnancy. This process continues past day 14.

Progesterone from the corpus luteum acts directly on the endometrium, causing arteries to enlarge. Glands in the uterus secrete nutrients into the uterine cavity. The cervical mucus becomes thick and tends to block sperm entry. The uterus is now ready to receive a fertilized egg.

If fertilization does not occur within about 24 hours of ovulation, the egg begins to disintegrate. The "no pregnancy" signal reaches the ovary, so the corpus luteum degenerates, and progesterone levels fall. The arteries of the endometrium begin to spasm and deprive the endometrial cells of oxygen and nutrients, so they die. The arteries constrict and then suddenly dilate. The sudden rush of blood causes capillary beds to disintegrate and causes the lining to detach from the uterine wall. The menstrual flow begins on about day 28. Figure 6.2 shows the changes in hormone levels, ovarian function, and uterine lining during a typical 28-day cycle.

PREGNANCY

If fertilization occurs, the zygote travels down the oviduct and enters the uterus. The embryo somehow signals the ovary that pregnancy has occurred. The corpus luteum is maintained and continues to secrete progesterone, which is essential to maintain the pregnancy. If progesterone levels fall or if the receptors in the uterus are blocked or ineffective, the uterus will contract and expel the lining and the embryo.

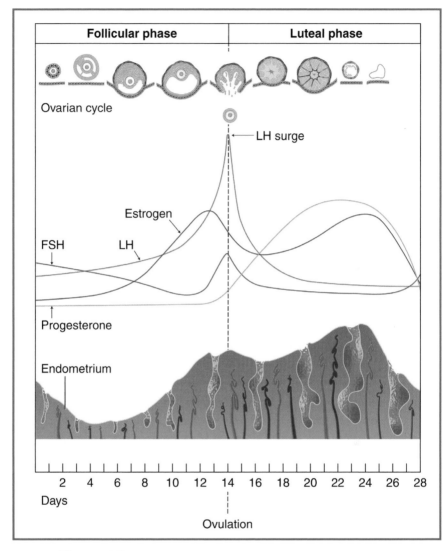

Figure 6.2 This diagram, illustrating the female reproductive cycle, shows what happens to the ovary, hormone levels, and uterine lining (endometrium) during a typical 28-day cycle. Day 1 is the start of the menstrual period. As the endometrium is shed, the pituitary gland releases FSH and LH, which stimulate the ovary to mature a new egg in its follicle. At day 14, ovulation occurs and the body prepares for pregnancy. If the egg is not fertilized, estrogen and progesterone levels drop and the cycle begins again.

Once the embryo enters the uterus and attaches to the uterine wall (implantation), several changes occur. The amounts of estrogen and progesterone increase throughout pregnancy. They are secreted by the ovary until the placenta is complete and takes over secretion at about week eight. Progesterone inhibits the release of prostaglandins, which cause uterine contractions and are probably involved in the onset of labor. Certain cells of the immune system involved with recognizing and destroying foreign tissue are also inhibited. This prevents the mother's immune system from detecting and destroying the developing embryo.

Two other hormones are secreted by the embryo and its early membranes. **Human chorionic gonadotropin** (HCG) is a **glycoprotein** that can be detected 6–8 days after ovulation by early pregnancy tests. Its primary action is to stimulate the corpus luteum to continue secreting progesterone. In addition, HCG appears to a have role in fetal development, especially the development of the testes in males. **Human placental lactogen** (hPL), another hormone secreted by the embryo, has lactogenic (milk-producing) and growth-hormone-like activity. It acts mainly on the maternal metabolism, apparently to ensure adequate nutrition for the fetus. Figure 6.3 shows the relative levels of the various hormones during a normal pregnancy.

During pregnancy, the mother's pituitary enlarges two to three times its normal size. Growth hormone, LH, and FSH levels are low, but another hormone, prolactin, is steadily rising. Throughout the pregnancy, estrogen inhibits prolactin release. Near the end of pregnancy, however, prolactin levels begin to increase, despite the presence of estrogen. Increased prolactin causes milk production to begin. In animals, prolactin is probably involved in certain maternal behaviors, such as "nesting behavior" in which mothers who are about to give birth try to find or build a place to house their young.

The signal to begin labor comes from the fetus. Although prostaglandins are involved somehow in labor, oxytocin is the

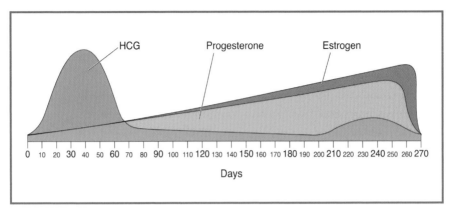

Figure 6.3 Hormone levels change during pregnancy, as seen in this graph. Human chorionic gonadotropin (HCG) is produced by the embryo until the placenta is mature enough to begin producing estrogen and progesterone. Early pregnancy tests measure HCG levels. At birth, the placenta is expelled, making hormone levels drop precipitously.

primary hormone during labor. Oxytocin is produced in the hypothalamus, stored in the pituitary, and released from the posterior pituitary under nervous stimulation from the hypothalamus. As the uterus contracts, nerve impulses travel up the spinal cord to the brain. The hypothalamus stimulates the pituitary to release more oxytocin and the uterine contractions get stronger. This cycle continues until the baby is born. The placenta is expelled soon after. Because the placenta has been the source of estrogen and progesterone for most of the pregnancy, the levels of both drop drastically after it is expelled. Suddenly, prolactin is no longer being inhibited, so true milk production begins shortly after giving birth. When the baby nurses, prolactin release is stimulated, which causes the milk supply to be maintained. Prolactin also inhibits the release of gonadotropins, so ovarian function decreases and, while she is nursing, a woman tends to not ovulate. However, within a few months of giving birth, most women return to their normal menstrual cycle.

CONNECTIONS

Male reproduction is controlled by a relatively simple negative feedback mechanism that maintains the levels of testosterone and sperm production once puberty has been reached. The loop includes the hypothalamus and the pituitary gonadotropin hormones just like female reproduction, but it lacks a monthly cycle.

The female reproductive process is more complicated because it includes a monthly cycle, and also provides means for becoming pregnant, maintaining the pregnancy, and producing milk to feed the infant. The hypothalamus stimulates the pituitary to release gonadotropins that bring

ENDOCRINE DISRUPTORS

Any chemical that can mimic, alter, or block the action of human hormones would be classified as an endocrine disruptor. Many naturally occurring plant compounds as well as synthetic chemicals are suspected of being able to change the development and reproduction of humans by disrupting normal estrogen and/or testosterone functions, typically by mimicking natural estrogens. Studies of wild animal populations as well as laboratory studies of cells and animals indicate that exposure to chemicals such as DES (diethylstilbestrol, a synthetic hormone), DDT (an insecticide widely used until it was banned in the 1970s), PCBs (polychlorinated biphenyls), and certain plastic products may cause serious health problems. For women, these "environmental estrogens" increase the risk of breast and reproductive tract cancer and endometriosis (the presence of uterine lining outside of the uterus). In males, these environmental chemicals cause reduced sperm counts and a high number of abnormal sperm as well as underdevelopment of the male reproductive organs. The full risks to humans and the environment are largely unknown and are controversial.

about the production of sex hormones and gametes. The ovaries and developing embryo produce estrogen, HCG, and progesterone, which sustain the actual pregnancy. The gender of the embryo is determined by the presence of either testosterone or estrogen. Oxytocin and prostaglandins initiate labor and delivery, and prolactin stimulates the production of milk.

7

Stress

Humans have two adrenal glands that are positioned on top of each kidney. Each gland, which is roughly shaped like a pyramid, weighs only 6–10 grams (0.2–0.35 ounces). If these glands were removed, a person would die within a few days. The adrenal glands help the body adjust and maintain itself through all the external and internal changes called stress. This maintenance process was first described by Walter B. Cannon (1871–1945), a physiologist at the Harvard School of Medicine. In 1926, he outlined the concept of homeostasis, in which the internal environment of the body is kept relatively constant. This has become the unifying concept in the physiology of all living things. In 1932, he described the relationship between the nervous system, stress, and the adrenal gland, and coined the term *fight-or-flight* to describe how the adrenal glands respond to emergency situations.

The concept of stress and the alarm reaction was developed by Hans Selye (1907–1982), a Hungarian physician who became professor and director of the Institute for Experimental Medicine and Surgery at the French University in Montreal. Selye called the body's response to stress the "**general adaptation syndrome.**" The idea was that animals (including humans) respond to stress and injury through a stereotypical series of nonspecific physiological responses that allow them to adapt or adjust to the situation and therefore avoid harm. This syndrome required the hypothalamus, pituitary, and the adrenal gland to work together.

Both Cannon and Selye described how the body responded to noxious situations, and both proved that the adrenal gland was essential to the response. However, the responses they described were very different. Cannon's fight-or-flight response takes place quickly (within seconds). The brain, heart, lungs, and muscles are almost immediately made ready for action. Selye's general adaptation syndrome takes much longer and produces changes in metabolism and overall physiology. In fact, both Cannon and Selye were correct. The structure of the adrenal gland itself explains how it can provide both a quick response and long-term changes.

During embryonic development, two different groups of cells migrate to the location of the kidney and join to form the adrenal glands (Figure 7.1). The cells that form the interior or medulla of the gland are of nervous origin. The cells that form the outer layer or cortex develop from the same kinds of cells that produce muscle and skeletal tissue. The two cell populations, and, therefore, the two layers of the adrenal glands, produce different groups of hormones that are controlled independently of each other. Cannon studied the medulla, and Selye studied the cortex.

THE ADRENAL MEDULLA

When a person is exposed to adverse conditions, such as cold, injury, danger, or fear, the brain takes in the information and processes it in various ways. The immediate response of the central nervous system is to release epinephrine and norepinephrine, which are also called adrenaline and noradrenaline, respectively. Epinephrine and norepinephrine, as well as other chemicals released by nerves, are collectively called neurotransmitters or transmitter substances. Their release can happen within milliseconds of the stimulus reaching the brain. Nerves send the chemicals to virtually all of the internal organs and even to the brain itself. The person is suddenly alert, the heart and breathing rates increase, and blood flow to the muscles increases. Nerve cells quickly run out of transmitter substances, however. After only a few minutes, the nervous system is unable to sustain the alert response.

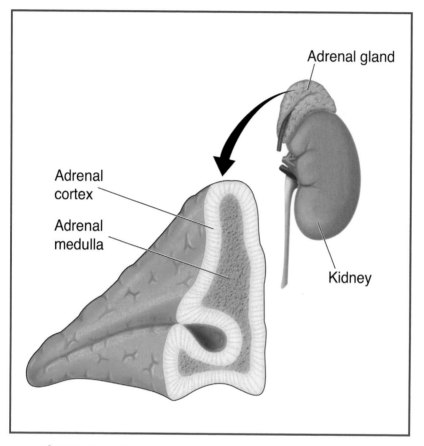

Figure 7.1 The shape and locations of the adrenal glands are shown here. The inner portion of the adrenal gland—the medulla—produces epinephrine, the fight-or-flight hormone. The outer portion—the cortex—produces a variety of steroids, including glucocorticoids, which raise blood glucose levels and suppress the immune system during times of stress.

Nerves run directly from the brain to the adrenal medulla. When the brain perceives a negative situation, these nerves stimulate the adrenal medulla to release epinephrine and norepinephrine. The adrenal gland produces exactly the same chemicals that the nervous system produced with exactly the same results. The primary difference is that the adrenals can continue to secrete the hormones for days. General physiological stresses, such as low oxygen or low blood glucose levels, also stimulate the adrenal medulla to release epinephrine.

EPINEPHRINE

Epinephrine and norepinephrine are similar molecules and have similar actions. They are both made from the amino acid tyrosine in certain nerve cells and in the adrenal medulla. Both hormones act on receptors called **adrenergic receptors** that are located throughout the body. The receptors are subdivided into two groups: alpha (α) and beta (β). Most organs have both types of receptors, but one type is usually predominant. Alpha receptors cause arteries to constrict, raising blood pressure. They also cause the muscles of the intestine to relax and the pupils to dilate. Beta receptors are much more common in the heart and the bronchial tubes of the lungs. Norepinephrine has a greater affinity for alpha receptors, and epinephrine is more likely to attach to beta receptors.

Each organ can respond to a particular situation in a different way depending on what type of receptors it has and whether it receives more epinephrine or norepinephrine. As a general rule, norepinephrine is more likely to be released by the nervous system, while the adrenal medulla releases about four times more epinephrine than norepinephrine. Table 7.1 shows the typical response to epinephrine by various body parts.

Epinephrine is the primary hormone released by the adrenal medulla in response to stress. As it circulates throughout the body, it causes the fight-or-flight response described by Cannon. The body prepares either to face the stress or run. The number of heartbeats per minute increases, and the contractions of the heart get stronger, pumping out more blood with each beat. The bronchioles of the lungs dilate, allowing more air into the lungs. Blood flow into the

Table 7.1 Organ Response to Epinephrine

Organ	Type of receptor	Response
Eye	α	Pupils dilate
Lungs	β	Bronchioles dilate
Heart	β	Rate increases
Digestive tract	α	Motility decreases
Liver	β	Glycogenolysis
Sweat glands	α	Secretion stimulated
Blood vessels in heart and muscles	β	Dilate
	α	Constrict
Adipose tissue	β	Lipolysis
Blood vessels in skin and gut	α	Constrict

Table 7.1 Receptors for epinephrine are called α or β adrenergic receptors. Which type of receptor an organ has determines how it will respond to the hormone.

lungs and to the muscles increases so that more oxygen is delivered to the muscles to allow them to do more work.

In the liver, epinephrine stimulates the breakdown of glycogen to glucose, thus raising blood glucose levels. The fat cells are stimulated to break down fat molecules and release fatty acids into the blood to be used as fuel, especially by muscle cells. A general increase in calorie usage occurs as more fuel is made available and as the body becomes more alert and active. The metabolic rate can increase by as much as 20–30%.

THE ADRENAL CORTEX

When stress continues for more than a few days, it is considered chronic. The adrenal medulla has helped the body to survive so far, but it cannot keep it alive without the adrenal cortex. The prolonged stress causes the brain to send a message to the hypothalamus, which, in turn, sends a signal to the anterior pituitary to release ACTH (adrenocorticotropic hormone). ACTH travels through the blood to the adrenal cortex and stimulates it to release glucocorticoids, primarily cortisol. ACTH is released several times a day, usually from 7 to 15 times, depending on the severity of the situation. Cortisol acts on the pituitary to decrease the amount of ACTH released. Figure 7.2 shows the pattern of control and feedback involved in cortisol release.

The adrenal cortex allows the body to maintain itself during long periods of physical or emotional stress, such as when a soldier is in combat or a person is starving. The cortex also allows the body to suppress the inflammation response that could cause swelling and pain and make escape more difficult. Suppressing the immune system can be a life-saving response in the short term, but for any length of time, it will have harmful effects, such as making the body more susceptible to disease-causing organisms (Figure 7.3).

EFFECTS OF CORTISOL ON THE METABOLISM
Glucocorticoids, including cortisol, act on several different tissues, such as muscle and liver cells, to make more fuel available for cells (Table 7.2). The net effect is to raise blood glucose levels. Many cells lower the amount of glucose they can transport across cell membranes, which leaves more glucose in the bloodstream and makes it available for brain and muscle cells to use. Protein molecules in muscle cells are broken down so that the amino acids can be sent to the liver. In the liver, the amino acids are converted into glucose, in the process called gluconeogenesis. Fat molecules are broken down to fatty acids and glycerol, which enter the blood and can be used as fuel by the liver and muscle cells.

When levels of cortisol remain high for prolonged periods of time, there are a number of adverse effects. Because of

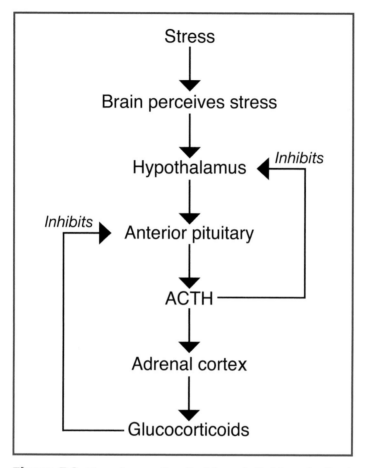

Figure 7.2 The relsease of cortisol is controlled by a feedback loop. Stress signals the hypothalamus, which alerts the anterior pituitary to release ACTH. ACTH then travels to the adrenal cortex, where it stimulates the release of glucocorticoids. When ACTH or glucocorticoid levels become too high, they reverse the process, inhibiting the release of hormone.

protein catabolism (breakdown), muscles become smaller and weaker. The skin gets thinner, and the protein matrix of bone can also decrease, causing bone formation to decrease. Less calcium is absorbed from the gut and more is lost in the urine, so bone density also decreases. Wounds heal more slowly

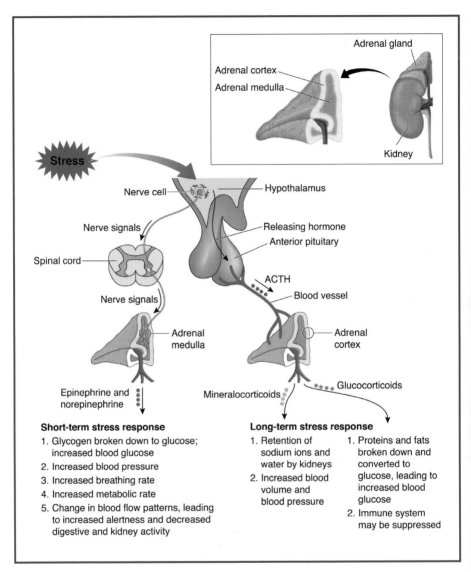

Figure 7.3 This diagram summarizes the responses of the adrenal glands to stress. The brain responds to physical and psychological stress by sending messages directly to the adrenal medulla to release epinephrine and norepinephrine to produce the fight-or-flight response. The hypothalamus also directs the pituitary to release adrenocorticotropic hormone (ACTH), which stimulates the adrenal cortex to release steroids that will increase blood volume, raise blood glucose levels, and suppress inflammation.

Table 7.2   Primary Actions of Adrenal Stress Hormones

Cortisol
- Increases
  - Fatty acid use
  - Protein breakdown
  - Gluconeogenesis
  - Stress resistance
  - Blood glucose
- Decreases
  - Inflammation
  - Wound healing speed
  - Use of glucose
- Regulates
  - Stress +
  - Glucocorticoid level –
  - Corticotropin-releasing hormone, ACTH +

Epinephrine and Norepinephrine
- Act quickly and briefly
- Fight-or-flight response
- Effects
  - Increase blood pressure
  - Increase cardiac output
  - Constrict peripheral blood vessels
  - Dilate most visceral blood vessels
  - Dilate bronchial tree
  - Decrease digestion
  - Increase muscle efficiency
  - Increase blood glucose
  - Increase cellular metabolism

Table 7.2 This table summarizes the actions of the steroid hormone cortisol and stress hormones epinephrine and norepinephrine.

than normal and bruising occurs more easily. Fat deposits are lost in the arms and legs and are deposited in the face, neck, and abdomen instead. In addition, the body retains more water. A person who is taking glucocorticoids, such as prednisone or cortisone, typically has a round, puffy face, called "moonface," caused by retention of excess fluid. If the excess glucocorticoids are produced by the body, the symptoms described above are collectively called Cushing's syndrome.

EFFECTS OF CORTISOL ON THE IMMUNE SYSTEM

Cortisol also affects the immune system by suppressing it. Usually, when a person is injured, the body has an inflammatory response in which the blood vessels in the injured area become leaky and white blood cells move toward the injury in response to chemical signals called **histamines** and prostaglandins. In addition, there will be redness and swelling at the site of injury.

During a period of prolonged stress, when cortisol is released, the hormone acts on the immune system in several ways. The hormone suppresses the release of histamines and prostaglandins and reduces the permeability of capillaries, thus decreasing local swelling. It suppresses the activity of many types of white blood cells, including the monocytes and macrophages that engulf and destroy invading organisms, such as bacteria, and stops the proliferation of lymphocytes. Cortisol suppresses the entire lymphatic system, and may cause lymph nodes to decrease in size. Some lymphocytes produce antibodies, proteins that are the first line of defense against invaders. If levels of cortisol are high enough, the number of antibodies in the blood can actually decrease.

Many bacteria make chemicals called toxins that actually produce the symptoms in the body. Cortisol blocks the effects of these toxins. For example, when patients with bacterial infections, such as pneumococcal pneumonia or tuberculosis, are given cortisol, the fever, toxin effects, and lung symptoms disappear. The bacteria are still alive in the patient's body, however, and will continue to spread if they are not killed with antibiotics. If a person is taking cortisone, it can actually cause a bacterial infection to go undetected until it is too late.

SURVIVAL VALUE

When a person is in danger, the adrenal medulla and cortex work together to maintain the body through the emergency and allow the person to get to safety. Epinephrine causes the brain to become alert, raises blood glucose levels, and increases blood flow to muscles. The adrenal cortex releases glucocorticoids (e.g., cortisol) that also raise blood glucose levels and suppress the immune system.

Raising blood glucose levels so that more fuel is available to muscle and brain cells helps the body survive and get out of the problem situation. For example, during a hike in the woods, if a person falls down a steep bank and sprains his or her ankle, epinephrine helps prepare the person for the exertion needed to climb up the bank to get help. As the person struggles up the bank and makes his or her way to the nearest emergency room, the cortisol released from the adrenal cortex keeps the ankle from swelling and allows the person to continue walking on it.

CONSEQUENCES OF STRESS

The brain does not distinguish between physical and mental stress. Long-term psychological or emotional stress, fear, anxiety, and apprehension will produce exactly the same physical response from the adrenal gland as physical danger does. Because the immune system is suppressed, people often become ill when they have been in stressful situations. For example, people who get cold sores, which are caused by a virus that lives inside nerve cells attached to the lips, usually get them when they are stressed physically by an infection, such as a cold. Emotional stress can also allow cold sores to appear, because the immune system is being suppressed in this situation as well. Without the stress, the immune system is able to keep the virus contained and no symptoms appear.

CONNECTIONS

The adrenal glands consist of two cell populations: the medulla and the cortex. Each part responds to different kinds of stress. The adrenal medulla, which responds to short-term stress, functions like part of the nervous system. It is controlled by nerves from the brain and releases epinephrine and norepinephrine, two chemicals that are also released by nerves. The result is called the fight-or-flight response. The adrenal cortex, which responds to chronic stress, produces steroids called glucocorticoids that raise blood glucose levels and decrease inflammation. The cortex is controlled by the hypothalamus and pituitary in response to chronic stress.

8

Hormones Maintain Mineral Balance and Blood Pressure

CALCIUM

An adult human body contains 2 to 3 pounds (0.9 to 1.4 kg) of calcium ions. Calcium is essential for many aspects of the human body, such as the strength of bones and teeth. Calcium ions (Ca^{+2}) join with phosphate ions ($PO4^{-3}$) to produce the hard mineral portion of the skeleton. Without calcium ions, blood will not clot adequately, nerve and muscle cells cannot function, and many hormones and enzymes will not work. To ensure the proper functioning of all these systems, the body regulates the level of calcium in the blood and other body fluids within very narrow limits (9–10.5 mg/100 ml of blood serum).

Three hormones are primarily responsible for regulating calcium metabolism. Parathyroid hormone (PTH) is secreted from the parathyroid glands, calcitonin is secreted from the thyroid gland, and a form of vitamin D called 1,25 dihydroxycholecalciferol or 1,25-dihydroxyvitamin D ($1,25\text{-}[OH]_2D$) is synthesized in the skin and activated in the liver and kidneys. The targets for these hormones are the bones, kidneys, and intestines. In general, PTH and vitamin D raise blood calcium levels, and calcitonin lowers them. Although PTH and vitamin D are essential for life, the body can apparently survive without calcitonin. This was first demonstrated during the 19th century when the thyroid was surgically removed to treat goiter. If the entire thyroid and the attached parathyroid glands were removed, the patient experienced severe muscle spasms and died.

Vitamin D is a steroid that is formed in a multistep process that begins in the skin when ultraviolet (UV) light acts on 7-dehydrocholesterol and converts it to cholecalciferol (vitamin D_3). Vitamin D_2, which is made by plants, is the form added to milk as a dietary supplement. Both vitamins D_2 and D_3 must be activated in the liver and then in the kidneys into the active form, 1,25-$(OH)_2D$, through a process controlled by PTH. Figure 8.1 shows the steps in this process.

BONE STRUCTURE

Bones are living, active, dynamic organs. They are made of a matrix of protein molecules with calcium salts embedded in them to make them hard. The minerals in bones are in a constant state of flux. The body may recycle as much as 5–7% of bone mass every week. The most solid part of our skeleton is actually completely replaced about every 10 years. Three types of bone cells live inside bone tissue. Osteocytes are mature bone cells that maintain the bone structure. Osteoclasts are large cells that dissolve bone and release calcium into the blood. Osteoblasts are bone-forming cells that take calcium out of the blood and store it in the bone. The activities of osteoblasts and osteoclasts are regulated by hormones. Figure 8.2 shows the microscopic structure of bone.

CALCIUM METABOLISM

Calcium ions are essential to the normal functioning of virtually all the cells in the body, so the concentration of Ca^{+2} in the blood must be carefully regulated. The cells of the parathyroid gland have calcium ion receptors on them. As blood calcium levels decrease, these cells respond

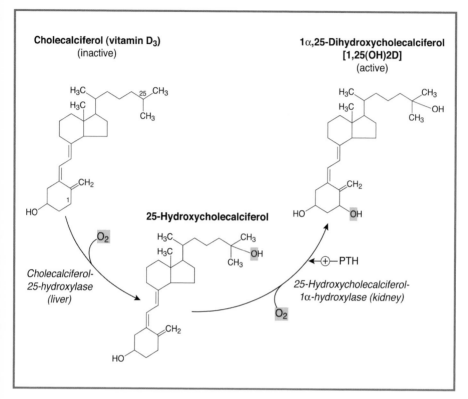

Figure 8.1 Activation of vitamin D is a two-step process. We ingest or synthesize the inactive form, which must then pass through the liver and kidney before it can have an effect on calcium metabolism.

by secreting PTH. If 1,25-(OH)$_2$D is present, osteocytes begin to release calcium from bone tissue within minutes. Osteoclasts are slower to respond to PTH, but they are much more efficient at removing calcium from the bones. PTH acts on the kidney and increases the reabsorption of calcium from the fluid in the kidney tubules to put calcium back into the blood instead of being excreted in the urine. At the same time, the activation of vitamin D described above is stimulated in the kidney.

There are two forms of vitamin D: inactive and active.

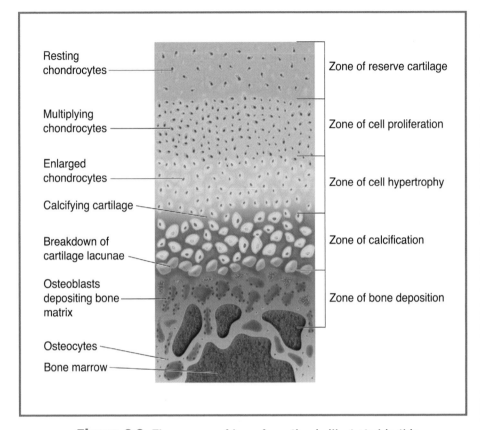

Resting chondrocytes

Multiplying chondrocytes

Enlarged chondrocytes

Calcifying cartilage

Breakdown of cartilage lacunae

Osteoblasts depositing bone matrix

Osteocytes

Bone marrow

Zone of reserve cartilage

Zone of cell proliferation

Zone of cell hypertrophy

Zone of calcification

Zone of bone deposition

Figure 8.2 The process of bone formation is illustrated in this diagram. Most of the bone in our body begins as cartilage that gradually changes into bone. Chondrocytes are cartilage cells. Osteoblasts produce bone, and osteocytes are mature bone cells. The process of changing cartilage into bone is called ossification. It requires large amounts of calcium and vitamin D.

Inactive vitamin D is acquired through foods or is made in the skin when it is exposed to ultraviolet light. Active vitamin D acts on the osteoclasts with PTH to increase the removal of calcium from bone and increase blood calcium levels. Vitamin D also acts on the lining of the small intestine and causes more calcium to be absorbed from the food being digested. If the calcium being removed from the bones is not replaced by calcium in the diet, the bones will weaken. For this reason, dietary recommendations for calcium are fairly high, from 400–1,500 mg per day, depending on age. As people get older, higher levels of calcium are recommended to prevent bone loss.

As blood calcium levels increase, less PTH is released. When blood calcium levels are higher than 9 mg/100 ml, the thyroid gland will begin to be secrete calcitonin. The primary action of calcitonin is to inhibit osteoclast activity, which allows the osteoblasts to activate and put calcium back into the bone tissue. As a result, blood calcium levels

YOUR HEALTH: OSTEOPOROSIS

Osteoporosis is a group of disorders in which bone is broken down faster than it is formed. The word comes from two Greek words: *osteon*, meaning "a bone," and *poros*, meaning "passage." When someone has osteoporosis, the bones become lighter, more porous, and weaker. The bones may become so weak, in fact, that the vertebrae may suffer compression fractures or the head of the femur may fracture (broken hip). Losing bone mass is a natural effect of aging, but it does not need to be debilitating. The worst effects of osteoporosis are avoidable. It is never too early to start preventing the condition, and it is never too late to reduce the symptoms.

Diet is key to reducing the risk of osteoporosis. Adequate levels of calcium and vitamin D, along with the other nutrients that are needed to form bone and other skeletal tissues (such as protein, vitamin C, and zinc), should be an important part of the diet. Fluoride helps build strong bones and teeth. Exercise also helps maintain strong bones. Bones respond to the stresses placed on them by becoming stronger, just as muscles do. And, like muscles, if bones are not used, they will become smaller and weaker. Load-bearing exercises such as lifting weights or gardening helps counter the effects of osteoporosis. Smoking and drinking alcohol have negative impacts on bone strength.

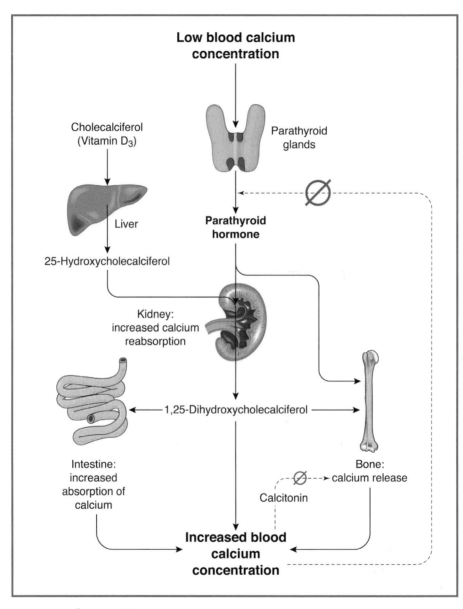

Figure 8.3 Parathyroid hormone (PTH) raises blood calcium levels by causing the kidney to increase the amount of active vitamin D. This, in turn, increases the amount of calcium absorbed from the intestine. Both vitamin D and PTH cause the bones to release stored calcium.

decrease. Figure 8.3 shows how these hormones work together to maintain calcium homeostasis.

Other hormones also have secondary effects on calcium metabolism because they affect bone growth and development. Testosterone and estrogen increase bone formation during childhood and puberty. Estrogen inhibits the bone resorption stimulated by PTH. It also facilitates the action of PTH on the kidney to activate vitamin D and to increase calcium reabsorption. In other words, estrogen protects the bones from calcium loss. The glucocorticoids (e.g., cortisol) from the adrenal cortex are necessary for normal bone formation, but if they are secreted in excess, they interfere with calcium absorption in the gut and kidney.

WATER AND ELECTROLYTE BALANCE

Humans are 60–65% water by weight. Water is found everywhere in the body: in the cells, surrounding the cells, in the blood plasma, in saliva, sweat, digestive juices, and urine. Dissolved in the water are a number of chemical substances called **electrolytes**. These are compounds that produce charged particles called ions that are capable of conducting electricity. The most important electrolytes are sodium (Na^+), potassium (K^+), magnesium (Mg^{+2}), and chloride (Cl^-). The individual and total concentrations of these ions in the blood are closely regulated, but none more so than sodium. Under normal circumstances, the concentration of sodium in blood plasma is about 140 mEq/L (milliequivalents per liter) and it varies less than 1%, despite wide fluctuations in consumption and excretion.

A number of systems and processes work together to control fluid and electrolyte homeostasis. When fluid levels are low or sodium too high, the brain signals the person that he or she is thirsty, so the person drinks. As a result, fluid levels increase and/or the sodium is diluted. The kidneys can conserve water and excrete salt, or they can save salt and excrete more water, depending on what the body needs. The cardiovascular system is involved in electrolyte balance because too much fluid in the blood vessels causes high blood pressure, or hypertension. High blood pressure can lead to heart attack, stroke, or kidney damage. Conversely, too little fluid will produce low blood pressure, which means the system cannot efficiently carry out its task of delivering oxygen and nutrients to cells and removing wastes. Low blood pressure can lead to tissue damage and fluid accumulation in the lungs and around the heart.

The electrolytes themselves are necessary for nerve impulses and muscle contraction. Ions are lost continuously in sweat, urine, and feces. If more electrolytes are excreted than are taken in, an electrolyte imbalance occurs. This imbalance can cause muscle cramps or spasms, dizziness, disorientation, and even coma and death. If the blood concentration becomes too great, during dehydration, for example, seizures and death can occur.

Several hormones work together to maintain normal water and electrolyte concentrations. They include antidiuretic hormone from the posterior pituitary, mineralocorticoids from the adrenal cortex, atrial natriuretic factor from the heart, and rennin-angiotensin from the kidneys. The organ that ultimately controls fluid and electrolyte balance is the kidney, so it is necessary to examine its structure and function to fully understand the process.

THE KIDNEY

Humans have two kidneys located in the back of the abdominal cavity at about the level of the waist (Figure 8.4). They are about four inches (10 cm) long and look much like their namesake, kidney beans. About 25% of the blood pumped out of the heart and into the aorta enters the kidneys through the renal arteries during periods of inactivity. The blood is then filtered, with the liquid portion and everything that is dissolved in it entering

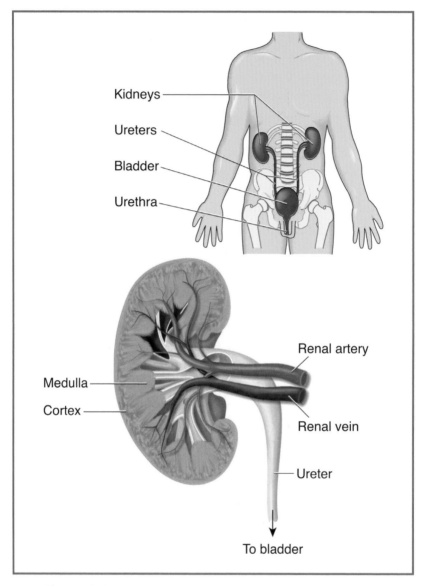

Figure 8.4 This diagram shows the structure and location of the kidneys. Humans have two kidneys attached to the back of the abdominal cavity at about waist level. Each kidney receives blood via a renal artery and releases it through a renal vein. The blood is filtered and water-soluble wastes are removed as urine. Urine travels down the ureters into the urinary bladder and exits through the urethra.

the million or so filtering units of the kidney, called **nephrons**. The fluid, now called filtrate, passes along a twisted tubule and is processed into urine. Substances the body requires, such as glucose, water, vitamins, and minerals, are returned to the blood, and waste products continue on within the tubule. The tubules send the urine into larger tubes called collecting ducts that lead to a funnel-shaped area of the kidney where the urine is collected before being sent to the urinary bladder.

On average, an adult's kidneys process about 180 liters of liquid per day, but excrete only about 1–1.5 liters of urine. At least 0.5 liter must be excreted every day to eliminate the water-soluble wastes from the body. This water must be replaced by eating or drinking to maintain the internal salt/water balance. The kidney can vary the volume and concentration of the urine depending on the body's needs and the levels of consumption of ions and water. Urine can be up to four times more concentrated than blood plasma or only one-fourth as concentrated. The hormones that control this process respond to different aspects of fluid balance and act on different parts of the kidney. This response allows the body to react quickly to changes in blood concentration, pressure, or volume.

ANTIDIURETIC HORMONE

In 1908, a German endocrinologist named Alfred Frank treated a man who had survived a gunshot to the head. The patient was always thirsty and urinated very frequently. An X-ray showed that the bullet had damaged the area of the skull that encloses the posterior portion of the pituitary. From this X-ray, Frank deduced that a hormone from the posterior pituitary must control water balance. This hormone came to be known as antidiuretic hormone (ADH), or vasopressin.

ADH is released from the posterior pituitary when receptors in the brain detect an increase in sodium concentration in the blood. Increased sodium concentration can be brought about by increased salt intake, dehydration, or loss of blood (hemorrhage). ADH acts primarily on the kidney to decrease urine output; hence, its name (*anti* means "against" and *diuresis* means "to urinate"). The specific targets within the kidney are the distal (far end) portion of the tubule and the collecting duct. The cells lining these portions of the nephrons become more permeable to water, so water leaves the tubules and collecting ducts and reenters the blood vessels. This lowers the volume and raises the concentration of the urine produced. Less water is excreted, so more returns to the bloodstream. As more water enters the bloodstream, the relative concentration of sodium is lowered, the receptors in the brain detect the change, and the secretion of ADH reduces. This is another example of a direct feedback loop, shown in Figure 8.5.

ADH secretion can also be affected by blood volume and cardiac output (how much blood is pumped out of the heart by each heartbeat). If blood volume is decreased by more than 8%, which is less than the pint of blood given by blood donors, or if cardiac output falls, ADH will be released. Increasing blood volume by saving water will help offset the blood loss and may increase cardiac output by simply increasing the volume of blood going into the heart. ADH also has a secondary action as a **vasoconstrictor** on blood vessels that serve the periphery (arms, legs, and external muscles of the trunk). Closing down the size of the arteries leading to these parts of the body increases blood pressure and tends to reroute blood to the essential body parts in the core of the body (brain and internal organs).

MINERALOCORTICOIDS

Mineralcorticoids are steroids secreted from the adrenal cortex, or outer layer of the adrenal gland, which affect electrolyte homeostasis. The main mineralocorticoid,

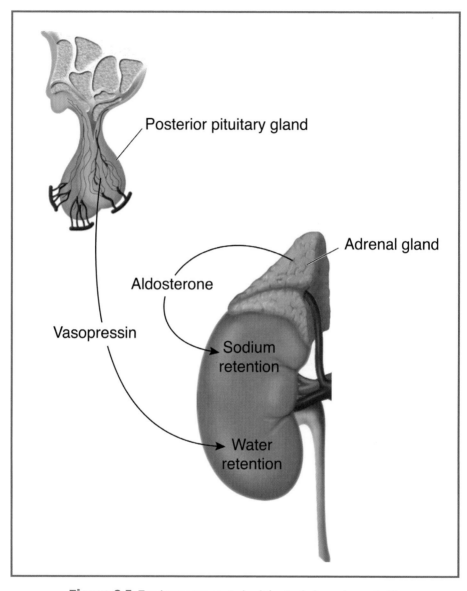

Posterior pituitary gland

Adrenal gland

Aldosterone

Vasopressin

Sodium retention

Water retention

Figure 8.5 Two hormones control salt/water balance by controlling urine output. Vasopressin is also called antidiuretic hormone (ADH). It is secreted by the pituitary in response to salt concentrations in the blood. It causes the kidney to save water and dilute salt. Aldosterone is a mineralocorticoid secreted by the adrenal cortex. It is also stimulates the kidney to retain water and salt.

aldosterone, is secreted primarily in response to decreased blood volume, but lowered sodium levels, elevated potassium levels, or reduced blood pressure can also trigger its release. Aldosterone acts on the distal tubules of the kidney nephrons, causing sodium to be reabsorbed into the blood. The reabsorption of sodium causes water to follow the sodium from the kidney tubules and enter the blood. The increase in sodium and water increases the blood volume, raising blood pressure. Aldosterone also increases the reabsorption of sodium in salivary and sweat glands as well as the large intestine.

The control of aldosterone release is not a simple system. It appears to be affected by a number of hormones besides

SPORTS DRINKS

During exercise, the body can lose large amounts of water and electrolytes in the form of sweat. In 1967, researchers at the University of Florida invented a mixture of water, sugar, and salts for the college's football team to drink. The researchers called the mixture Gatorade®, after the schools' team name, the Gators. It worked better than water to keep the players hydrated. That year, the Gators won their first-ever Orange Bowl. Today, grocery store aisles are filled with sports drinks. Do they work?

Research has shown that if a person exercises for one hour or more, he or she should probably have a sports drink. The sugar from the drink provides energy, and the salts replace electrolytes that have been lost. However, the biggest advantage is that sports drinks are better able to replace the water lost than plain water is. Adult athletes ingest a larger volume of liquid when they drink flavored drinks. In tests done with children, the presence of the flavor and the electrolytes together were important in getting test subjects to drink enough to replace what they had lost during activity. The extras available in many the actual sodium concentration of the blood. Adreno-corticotropic hormone (ACTH), which is released from the pituitary during periods of stress, has some effect on aldosterone release, but is apparently not required. **Angiotensin** from the kidney (described in the next section) also increases aldosterone secretion. Elevated blood potassium levels increase aldosterone secretion, and one of the secondary effects of aldosterone is to increase excretion of potassium by the kidney. In fact, the result of too much aldosterone is hypertension accompanied by potassium depletion called **hypokalemia.**

At first glance, it may appear that aldosterone and ADH are redundant hormones. In actuality, they complement

sports drinks, however, such as choline, creatine, or vitamins, are not really worth the added expense for most people.

The National Athletic Trainers' Association recommends that 17–20 ounces (about half a liter) of liquid be ingested at least one hour before activity, and another 7–10 ounces (about a quarter of a liter) just before exercise. They also recommend that athletes take drink breaks every 45 minutes during exercise and then drink another 28 to 40 ounces (0.83 to 1.2 liters) after exercise. It is also recommended that, after exercising, athletes drink 20 ounces (0.6 liters) of liquid for each pound (0.45 kg) of weight lost during exercise. The amount of weight lost during exercise varies from person to person, but as an example, an adult male baseball player playing a full game on a hot day can lose up to 10 pounds (4.5 kg).

The bottom line is that if a person exercises strenuously for extended periods of time, a sports drink may help the person's performance and increase endurance because the person will be better hydrated, especially in warm environments. If the person is active for less than one hour or is only doing light exercise, plain water will be just as effective for hydration.

each other. ADH responds primarily to blood concentration, whereas aldosterone responds to blood volume. Blood concentration may be affected without altering blood volume and, conversely, the blood volume may fall without changing electrolyte concentrations, as would occur during hemorrhage.

RENIN-ANGIOTENSIN SYSTEM

Certain cells located at the beginning of each nephron are sensitive to blood pressure. When blood pressure falls, the cells release a hormone called **renin** into the bloodstream. Renin acts on a protein made by the liver and present in the blood called angiotensinogen, converting it into angiotensin I. Angiotensin I is quickly converted by various body tissues into angiotensin II, a potent vasoconstrictor. The constriction of arteries quickly raises blood pressure, and the kidney cells respond by reducing the secretion of renin.

Angiotensin II has two secondary actions. It acts on the brain to induce drinking behavior (it makes us thirsty). It also stimulates the release of aldosterone, which increases blood volume and therefore blood pressure. Angiotensin II is not normally present in most people, but it is found in people who suffer from what is called **essential hypertension**, when the primary cause of the elevated blood pressure is not known. Figure 8.6 shows the relationships of the **renin-angiotensin** system.

ATRIAL NATRIURETIC FACTORS

The human heart has four chambers. The upper chambers, called atria, receive blood. The lower two chambers, called ventricles, pump the blood. The right side of the heart receives the blood from the body that is low in oxygen and sends it to the lungs, where the blood becomes oxygenated. The oxygenated blood returns to the left side of the heart and

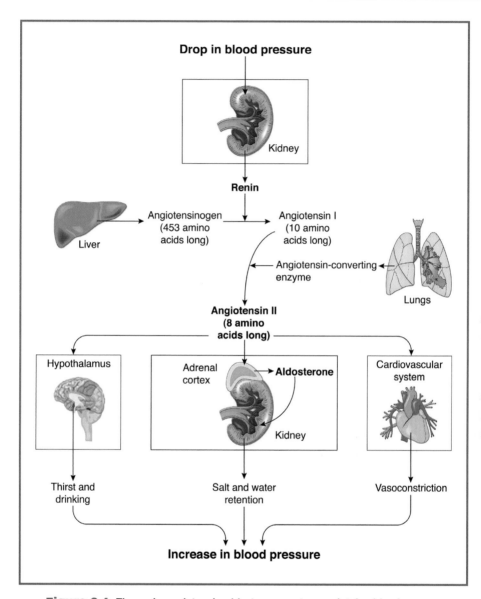

Figure 8.6 The renin-angiotensin-aldosterone system maintains blood pressure. When blood pressure decreases, the kidneys secrete renin, which converts angiotensinogen to angiotensin I. Angiotensin I is then converted to angiotensin II. This hormone acts on the brain to produce thirst, on the adrenal cortex to release aldosterone, and also constricts arteries. Increasing the amount of water in the blood raises blood volume. This, along with the narrowing of the arteries, raises blood pressure.

is then pumped out of the left ventricle into the aorta and then to the body.

When pressure increases in the right atrium, a group of peptides called atrial natriuretic factors (ANF) are released by cells in the wall of the atrium. These factors stimulate the kidney to produce more urine (diuresis), which then reduces fluid volume in the body and, therefore, blood pressure. The net effect is to counteract and inhibit ADH, aldosterone, and renin.

ANF works on several sites within the kidney, but primarily on the tubules of the nephron to keep electrolytes within the tubule. This effect causes more sodium to be excreted, which accounts for the name—*natriuretic*—which means "sodium excretion." (The chemical symbol for sodium is Na, which comes from its Latin name, *natrium*.) Renin secretion is inhibited because ANF increases the blood pressure in the vessels that signal its release.

ANF also acts on several other parts of the body. In the cardiovascular system, it lowers blood pressure directly by dilating arteries and reducing cardiac output. Secretion of aldosterone by the adrenal glands is inhibited. The central nervous system is affected in two ways: Water and salt appetites are decreased and the release of ADH is inhibited.

CONNECTIONS

There are many ions dissolved in the blood plasma whose concentrations are maintained within narrow limits. Calcium is necessary for strong bones and teeth as well as nerve impulse conduction, muscle contractions, and blood clotting. Sodium is also needed for nerve impulses and muscle contractions. The relative amounts of water and sodium are regulated by the interactions of several hormones that work on the nervous, cardiovascular, and urinary systems. Antidiuretic hormone, aldosterone, renin, angiotensin, and atrial natriuretic factor work together to

Table 8.1 Summary of Actions of Hormones That Affect Blood Pressure and Urine Output

	ANF	Angiotensin II	ADH	Aldosterone
Behavior				
Drink water	-	+		
Eat salt	-			
Hypothalamus				
ADH release	-		-	
Kidney				
Urine output	+		-	-
Salt excretion	+		-	-
Renin release	-			
Adrenal				
Aldosterone secretion	-	+		
Cardiovascular system				
Blood volume	-	+	+	+

Table 8.1 Atrial natriuretic factor (ANF) lowers blood pressure by inhibiting the hormones and behaviors that raise it and by increasing urine output. Angiotensin II, ADH (antidiuretic hormone), and aldosterone all raise blood pressure by increasing blood volume.

maintain a nearly constant blood volume with a constant concentration of ions dissolved in it. A summary of actions of hormones that affect blood pressure and urine output are shown in Table 8.1.

Glossary

Acromegaly Disease caused by excess growth hormone in adults. It results in enlarged fingers, ears, and nose.

Adenylate cyclase An enzyme that converts ATP to cAMP as part of a signal pathway.

Adrenal cortex Outer layer of adrenal gland. Produces steroid hormones including glucocorticoids like cortisone, and mineralocorticoids like aldosterone.

Adrenaline *See* **Epinephrine.**

Adrenal medulla Inner layer of adrenal gland. Produces epinephrine and norepinephrine.

Adrenergic receptors Receptors for epinephrine (adrenaline). The binding of epinephrine to the receptor causes a reaction within the cell.

Adrenocorticotropic hormone (**ACTH**) Pituitary hormone that stimulates adrenal cortex to release steroids.

Age-onset diabetes *See* **Non-insulin-dependent diabetes mellitus.**

Aldosterone Steroid hormone from adrenal medulla. Stimulates kidneys to reabsorb sodium ions (Na^+), which increases water reabsorption and reduces urine production.

Amines Chemicals with an amine group ($-NH_2$); include amino acids and their derivatives.

Anabolic Production of large molecules; synthesis, especially of protein.

Androgens Male sex hormones.

Angiotensin Either of two forms of the hormone kinin that acts as a vasoconstrictor.

Antidiuretic hormone (**ADH**) Pituitary hormone that stimulates kidney to save water by reducing urine output.

Atrial natriuretic factor (**ANF**) Hormone produced by specialized cells within the heart that increases water loss through the kidneys and reduces blood pressure.

Basal metabolic rate (BSM) The amount of energy needed to maintain an organism at rest.

Calcitonin Thyroid hormone that reduces blood calcium levels.

cAMP Cyclic adenosine monophosphate.

Carbohydrate Sugars and large molecules made of sugars (starch, fiber).

Cascade Series of steps that amplifies a response.

Corticosteroid Any of four groups of steroids excreted by the adrenal gland.

Cretinism A form of mental retardation caused by lack of thyroid hormone during development or early childhood.

Diabetes mellitus Disease caused by insufficient insulin or lack of response to insulin resulting in elevated blood glucose levels.

Dwarfism A condition in which growth hormone deficiency (GHD) causes a person to be abnormally short.

Electrolytes Substances that dissolve in water and produce charged particles that conduct electricity.

Endocrine gland Ductless gland that secretes hormones into blood.

Endocrine system The ductless glands and the hormones they secrete that work with the nervous system to maintain the body.

Endorphins Naturally occurring painkilling chemicals found in the central nervous system.

Epinephrine Hormone released by adrenal medulla and by nervous system. Produces fight-or-flight response.

Essential hypertension Condition of elevated blood pressure for which the primary cause is unknown.

Estrogens Female sex hormones.

Fight-or-flight response Nervous and/or endocrine response to stress. Epinephrine is released, resulting in increased heart and respiration rates.

Glossary

Follicle stimulating hormone (FSH) Pituitary hormone that stimulates gonads to produce gametes.

General adaptation syndrome Another name for the fight-or-flight response.

Gestational diabetes Diabetes that only occurs during pregnancy due to increased resistance to insulin.

Gigantism Condition in which excess growth hormone is produced before the bones stop growing, causing a person to be abnormally tall.

Glucocorticoids Steroid hormones produced by the adrenal cortex that regulate blood glucose levels and inhibit the immune system.

Gluconeogenesis Producing glucose from noncarbohydrate sources, such as amino acids.

Glycogen Branched polymer of glucose stored in liver and muscles; short-term energy storage.

Glycogenesis Production of glycogen, the short-term energy storage carbohydrate found in liver and muscle.

Glycogenolysis Breaking glycogen down to glucose.

Glycoprotein A type of protein that includes a nonprotein group that is a carbohydrate.

Goiter Enlargement of the thyroid gland.

Gonadotropin releasing hormone (GnRH) Controlling hormone released by hypothalamus. Stimulates release of FSH and LH from pituitary.

Gonadotropins Hormones that stimulate the gonads (ovaries and testes) to produce gametes and hormones.

Gonads The sex organs—ovaries and testes.

G protein Protein on cell membrane that is intermediary in signal transduction process.

Graves' disease A condition caused by over-secretion of thyroid hormone; results in elevated metabolic rate, loss of weight, and often protruding eyes.

Growth hormone Pituitary hormone that stimulates tissue growth.

Histamines Chemicals released by damaged cells that increase blood flow to area.

Homeostasis Dynamic maintenance of a constant internal environment.

Hormone Specific chemical signal that is produced in one part of the body and travels through the blood to another part of the body, where it has a specific action.

Human chorionic gonadotropin (HCG) Hormone released during early stages of pregnancy.

Human placental lactogen (hPL) Hormone produced by the placenta that stimulates the mammary gland to produce milk.

Hydrophilic Water-loving; substances that dissolve in water.

Hydrophobic Water-hating; substances that do not dissolve in water.

Hyperglycemic When blood glucose levels are higher than normal.

Hyperthyroidism Condition caused by oversecretion of thyroid hormone.

Hypoglycemic When blood glucose levels are lower than normal.

Hypokalemia A condition in which blood potassium levels are too low.

Hypophyseal portal Special bed of capillaries that connects the hypothalamus directly to the pituitary.

Hypophysis Another name for the pituitary gland; from the Greek for "to grow under."

Hypothalamus Region of the brain that maintains homeostasis.

Hypothermia A condition in which body temperature decreases significantly below normal.

Hypothyroidism Condition caused by insufficient secretion of thyroid hormone.

Insulin Hormone from the pancreas that lowers blood glucose levels by increasing uptake by cells.

Glossary

Insulin-dependent diabetes mellitus (IDDM) Also known as type 1 or juvenile-onset diabetes; a form of diabetes caused by the destruction of a person's islet cells by his or her own immune system. This condition is usually treated with insulin injections.

Islets of Langerhans Specialized cells in the pancreas that produce insulin and glucagon.

Juvenile-onset diabetes *See* **Insulin-dependent diabetes mellitus.**

Ketoacidosis Lowered blood pH due to a buildup of ketone bodies. Typically occurs during starvation, uncontrolled diabetes, and high fat and protein diets.

Lipids Family of organic compounds, including fats, waxes, and steroids, that are not water-soluble.

Lipogenesis Fat synthesis.

Lipolysis Process of breaking down fats to utilize them as an energy source.

Luteinizing hormone (LH) Gonadotropin from the pituitary gland that stimulates ovulation in females and testosterone production in males.

Lymphocytes White blood cells.

Melanocyte stimulating hormone (MSH) A hormone that may play a role in the metabolism of fat.

Melatonin Hormone released from the pineal gland.

Mineralocorticoids Steroids released from the adrenal cortex that regulate salt/water balance.

Mucopolysaccharides Large molecules made of sugar and protein.

Nephrons Functional unit of the kidney.

Nervous system The brain, spinal cord, and nerves.

Neurotransmitters Chemical signals released from the terminal of one nerve cell that stimulate the next nerve cell.

Non-insulin-dependent diabetes mellitus (NIDDM) Also known as type 2 diabetes or age-onset diabetes; condition when the release of insulin is decreased or irregular, or insulin receptors have reduced sensitivity.

Nonpolar Having no polar regions. Molecules of this type do not dissolve in water.

Noradrenaline *See* **Norepinephrine.**

Norepinephrine Hormone released from adrenal medulla in response to stress. Also called noradrenaline.

Oxytocin Hormone released from the hypothalamus that causes uterine contractions.

Parathyroid gland Four endocrine glands attached to the back of the thyroid gland that secrete parathyroid hormone, which raises blood calcium levels.

Phospholipids Molecules that make up the cell membranes. They consist of a polar hydrophilic head and a nonpolar, hydrophobic tail.

Pineal gland Small endocrine structure in the brain that produces melatonin; regulates seasonal behavior.

Pituitary gland Small structure located on ventral surface of the brain. It is controlled by the hypothalamus and controls many other endocrine glands.

Polar Containing charged areas; polar chemicals dissolve in water.

Progesterone Steroid hormone that is produced by the ovaries and maintains pregnancy.

Prolactin Pituitary hormone that stimulates milk production.

Proteins Polymers made of amino acids. They serve as catalysts, structural components, and nutritional components.

Proteogenesis The synthesis of protein.

Renin Hormone secreted by kidneys when blood pressure or blood flow decreases. Converts angiotensinogen to angiotensin I.

Glossary

Renin-angiotensin system Complex hormone system that regulates salt/water balance and blood pressure.

Seasonal affective disorder (SAD) Disorder caused by lack of daylight; one of the symptoms is lethargy.

Sex hormones Estrogen, progesterone, and testosterone; the steroids that produce sexual characteristics.

Signal transduction A mechanism that links mechanical or chemical signals to specific cellular responses.

Somatostatin Chemical released by the hypothalamus that inhibits the release of growth hormone.

Somatotrophin Another name for growth hormone.

Steroids Lipid chemicals derived from cholesterol; they include the sex hormones and adrenocorticoid hormones.

Sterol Another name for a steroid.

Synergist Something that assists.

Target cells Cells that respond to specific hormones.

Testosterone Male sex hormone.

Tetraiodothyronine One of the three hormones excreted by the thyroid gland (T_4); also known as thyroxine.

Thymosin A chemical that activates the lymphocytes of the immune system.

Thymus Endocrine gland located in neck; establishes and activates the immune system.

Thyroid stimulating hormone (TSH) Controlling hormone released by pituitary that stimulates the thyroid gland to release thyroid hormone.

Thyroxine Another name for tetraiodothyronine, one of the three thyroid hormones.

Triiodothyronine One of the three hormones excreted by the thyroid gland. (T_3).

Type 1 diabetes   See **Insulin-dependent diabetes mellitus.**

Type 2 diabetes   See **Non-insulin-dependent diabetes mellitus.**

Tyrosine   Amino acid; precursor of thyroid hormones.

Vasoconstrictor   Substance that causes arteries to constrict, increasing blood pressure.

Bibliography

American Diabetes Association. *American Diabetes Association Complete Guide to Diabetes*, 2nd ed. New York: Bantam Books, 1999.

Bailey, Sue. "Insulin: A Canadian medical miracle of the 20th century." *The Canadian Press*, 2003. Available online at *http://www.ch1.ca/ CANOE2000/health_1.html*.

Becker, Wayne M., Lewis J. Kleinsmith, and Jeff Hardin. *The World of the Cell*, 5th ed. San Francisco: Benjamin Cummings, 2003.

Beckman, Joshua A., Mark A. Creager, and Peter Libby. "Diabetes and Atherosclerosis: Epidemiology, Pathophysiology, and Management." *Journal of the American Medical Association* 287 (19) (2002): 2570–2579.

Breslau, Neil A. "Calcium Homeostasis." *Textbook of Endocrine Physiology*, eds. James E. Griffin and Sergio R. Ojeda. New York: Oxford University Press, 1996.

Campbell, Neil A., and Jane B. Reece. *Biology*, 6th ed. San Francisco: Benjamin Cummings, 2002.

Cohen, Pinchas, and Ron G. Rosenfeld. "Growth Regulation." *Textbook of Endocrine Physiology*, eds. James E. Griffin and Sergio R. Ojeda. New York: Oxford University Press, 1996.

Friedrich, M.J. "Causes Sought for Neural Tube Defects in Infants of Diabetic Pregnant Women." *Journal of the American Medical Association* 287 (19) (2002): 2487–2488.

Ganang, William F. *Review of Medical Physiology*, 17th ed. Norwalk, CT: Appleton & Lange, 1995.

Griffin, James E. "The Thyroid." *Textbook of Endocrine Physiology*, eds. James E. Griffin and Sergio R. Ojeda. New York: Oxford University Press, 1996.

Griffin, James E., and Sergio R. Ojeda, eds. *Textbook of Endocrine Physiology*. New York: Oxford University Press, 1996.

Kaplan, Norman M. "The Adrenal Glands." *Textbook of Endocrine Physiology*, eds. James E. Griffin and Sergio R. Ojeda. New York: Oxford University Press, 1996.

Mader, Sylvia. *Biology*, 8th ed. New York: McGraw-Hill, 2004.

Marieb, Elaine N. *Human Anatomy & Physiology*, 5th ed. San Francisco: Benjamin Cummings, 2001.

McCracken, Joan, and Donna Hoel. "From ants to analogues: Puzzles and promises in diabetes management." *Postgraduate Medicine* 101 (4) (1997): 138.

McKee, Trudy, and James R. McKee. *Biochemistry: An Introduction.* Boston: McGraw-Hill, 1999.

Medvei, Victor C. *A History of Endocrinology.* Lancaster, UK: MTP Press, 1982.

Pagana, Kathleen Deska, and Timothy James Pagana. *Mosby's Diagnostic and Laboratory Test Reference*, 2nd ed. St. Louis: Mosby-Year Book, Inc., 1995.

Stewart, Kerry J. "Exercise training and the Cardiovascular Consequences of Type 2 Diabetes and Hypertension." *Journal of the American Medical Association* 288 (13) (2002): 1622–1631.

Surks, Martin I. *The Thyroid Book.* Yonkers, NY: Consumers Union, 1993.

Turner, C. Donnell, and Joseph T. Bagnara. *General Endocrinology.* Philadelphia: W.B. Saunders, 1971.

"The Way We Live Now: 3-16-03: The Body Check; The Bittersweet Science." *The New York Times.* March 16, 2003, Sec. 6, p. 18.

Voet, Donald, and Judith G. Voet. *Biochemistry*, 2nd ed. New York: John Wiley & Sons, 1995.

Wilk, B., and O. Bar-Or. "Effect of drink flavor and NaCl on voluntary drinking and hydration in boys exercising in heat." *Journal of Applied Physiology* 80 (4) (1996): 1112–1117.

World Health Organization. "Micronutrient deficiencies." September 12, 2002. Available online at *http://who.int/nut/idd.htm.*

Websites

American Diabetes Association
www.diabetes.org

American Foundation of Thyroid Patients
www.thyroidfoundation.org

Calcium Information Resources
www.calciuminfo.com

Centers for Disease Control and Prevention
www.cdc.gov

Diabetes—News From Medical Journals
www.diabetes.com

e.hormone, Tulane University
http://e.hormone.tulane.edu

Gatorade®
www.gatorade.com

The History of Insulin
www.med.uni-giessen.de/itr/history/inshist.html

The Hormone Foundation,
The Public Education Affiliate of the Endocrine Society
www.hormone.org

Human Growth Foundation
www.hgfound.org

MEDLINEplus Medical Encyclopedia
www.medlineplus.gov

National Athletic Trainers' Association
www.nata.org

National Diabetes Information Clearinghouse
http://diabetes.niddk.nih.gov/

National Institute of Health. Environmental Health Perspectives.
Phytoestrogens: friends or foes?
http://Ehpnet1.niehs.nih.gov/docs/1996/104-5/focus.html

Bilezikian, John P., et al. *The Parathyroids: Basic and Clinical Concepts.* New York: Raven Press, 1994.

Pierpaoli, Walter, William Regelson, and Carol Colman. *The Melatonin Miracle.* New York: Simon & Schuster, 1995.

Rosen, Clifford J. "Restoring Aging Bones." *Scientific American.* March 2003, pp. 71–77.

Appendix

INFORMATION ON STEROID USE AND ABUSE

American College of Sports Medicine

www.acsm.org

ATHENA (Athletes Targeting Health Exercise and Nutrition
Alternatives) for Young Female Athletes

www.ohsu.edu/hpsm/athena.html

ATLAS (Athletes Learning to Avoid Steroids)
for Young Male Athletes

www.ohsu.edu/hpsm/atlas.html

National Institute on Drug Abuse InfoFacts

www.drugabuse/gov/Infofax/steroids.html

National Institute on Drug Abuse Research Reports Series

www.drugabuse.gov/ResearchReports/Steroids/anabolicsteroid2.html

Unit (metric)		Metric to English	English to Metric	
LENGTH				
Kilometer	km	1 km 0.62 mile (mi)	1 mile (mi)	1.609 km
Meter	m	1 m 3.28 feet (ft)	1 foot (ft)	0.305 m
Centimeter	cm	1 cm 0.394 inches (in)	1 inch (in)	2.54 cm
Millimeter	mm	1 mm 0.039 inches (in)	1 inch (in)	25.4 mm
Micrometer	µm			
WEIGHT (MASS)				
Kilogram	kg	1 kg 2.2 pounds (lbs)	1 pound (lbs)	0.454 kg
Gram	g	1 g 0.035 ounces (oz)	1 ounce (oz)	28.35 g
Milligram	mg			
Microgram	µg			
VOLUME				
Liter	L	1 L 1.06 quarts	1 gallon (gal)	3.785 L
			1 quart (qt)	0.94 L
			1 pint (pt)	0.47 L
Milliliter	mL or cc	1 mL 0.034 fluid ounce (fl oz)	1 fluid ounce (fl oz)	29.57 mL
Microliter	µL			
TEMPERATURE				
$°C = 5/9 \ (°F - 32)$		$°F = 9/5 \ (°C + 32)$		

Index

Index

Index

Picture Credits

About the Author

Lynette Rushton is a native of Washington State. She is a Professor of Biology and Chemistry at South Puget Sound Community College in Olympia, WA. She has been a full-time faculty member at SPSCC since 1992 and is listed in Who's Who Among America's College Teachers. She received a Bachelor of Science degree in Zoology from the University of Washington in Seattle, Washington. As an undergraduate, her studies focused on vertebrate anatomy and physiology. As a graduate student, she worked primarily on the endocrinology of reproduction in mammals. She received a Masters of Science in Biology from Eastern Washington University in Cheney, Washington.